Thank you for your
encouragement and support

Pauline

Mental Health and Politics in Northern Ireland

A history of service development

PAULINE PRIOR

Avebury

Aldershot · Brookfield USA · Hong Kong · Singapore · Sydney

Published by
Avebury
Ashgate Publishing Limited
Gower House
Croft Road
Aldershot
Hants GU11 3HR
England

Ashgate Publishing Company
Old Post Road
Brookfield
Vermont 05036
USA

British Library Cataloguing in Publication Data

Prior, Pauline M.
    Mental Health and Politics in Northern Ireland:
    History of Service Development
    I. Title
    362.209416

ISBN 1 85628 540 5

Copyright for maps: for permission to reproduce the maps on page xii the author acknowledges Harkness, D. (1983) *Northern Ireland since 1920.* Dublin: Helicon Ltd.

Typeset by
Textflow Services Limited
The Science Library
Lennoxvale
Belfast BT9 5EQ

Printed and Bound in Great Britain by
Athenaeum Press Ltd, Newcastle upon Tyne.

Figures and tables

Acknowledgements

As the research for this book began in 1985, it would be impossible to name all of the people who have helped me. However, special thanks are due to the following people: Professor Kathleen Jones and Professor Jonathan Bradshaw of the University of York; Dr Arthur Williamson and Professor Derek Birrell of the University of Ulster; the staff of Queen's University Medical Library, especially Jean O'Connor, Sean O'Brien and Anne Marie Bogle; the staff of the Public Record Office (NI); Jim Smyth and Brenda Quinn of the Eastern Health and Social Services Board; Dr Jim Jamison, Stanley Herron and Pat McGrew of the DHSS(NI); Dr Michael Donnelly and Pat McEvoy of the Health and Health Care Research Unit, Belfast; Jan Maconaghie, Assistant Director Social Services and my colleagues on the Social Services Training Team of the Northern Health and Social Services Board; Renee Boyd, formerly Principal Social Worker (Health Care) in North and West Belfast; and Dr Art O'Connor of The Central Mental Hospital, Dublin. I would also like to say thanks to the patients who shared their experiences with me and whose names I cannot mention. My final thanks for editorial comments and psychological support go to Tina Davis, Nina Oldfield and Dai Griffiths.

Abbreviations

CPN	Community psychiatric nurse
DHSS	Department of Health and Social Services
ECT	Electro convulsive therapy
HPSS	Health and Personal Social Services
IRA	Irish Republican Army
ITO	Industrial Therapy Organisation
NAMH	National Association for Mental Health
NI	Northern Ireland
NIA	Northern Ireland Assembly
NIAMH	Northern Ireland Association for Mental Health
NICRA	Northern Ireland Civil Rights Movement
NIO	Northern Ireland Office
NIHA	Northern Ireland Hospitals Authority
PRO(NI)	Public Record Office for Northern Ireland
QUB	The Queen's University of Belfast
ROI	Republic of Ireland
RUC	Royal Ulster Constabulary

**Lunatics abound more in Ulster
than any other part of Ireland**

*William Todd,
Secretary of the Asylum Commission 1819.*

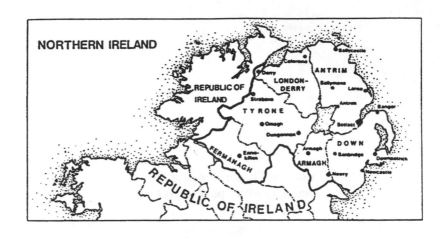

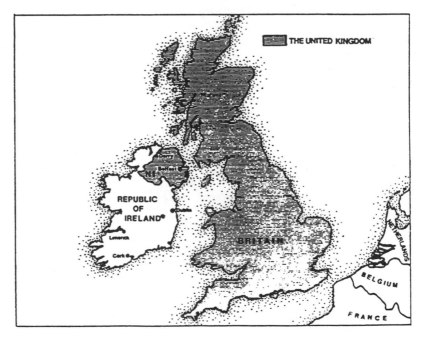

Source: *Harkness 1983*

Introduction

Northern Ireland, because it is a divided and troubled society, provides a unique environment for the study of social issues. Needs and solutions are thrown into sharp relief by the volatile nature of the political environment which has changed repeatedly since 1921. Unlike other areas of social provision such as education, housing and employment, health policy has not been a focus for research. This study is concerned with the relationship between political factors and mental health service developments since the establishment of Northern Ireland as a political entity in 1921. The questions addressed include the following: How did the lunacy services of the nineteenth century evolve into a modern mental health care system? How adequate have the services been over time? How did the legal context for these services change? How did the political context within which policy decisions were being made affect the direction of policy change? And finally, were internal factors more (or less) influential than external factors in policy formation and implementation?

In Chapter One, the pattern of services and legislation inherited from the nineteenth century are examined in the context of a newly emerging Northern Ireland. Reasons for the lack of development in any aspect of mental health policy are explored, to determine the main factors causing stagnation. In Chapter Two, the introduction of the Mental Treatment Act (NI) 1932 is analysed. A complex legal system for hospital admission, based on at least nine different pieces of nineteenth century lunacy law, was replaced by a simple legal framework for hospital treatment. The focus of this chapter is not confined to the content of the law, but extends to the fundamental issues of policy initiation and formulation. Chapter Three illustrates the impact of political developments in Britain on mental health policy in Northern Ireland. The introduction of a national health service structure throughout the United Kingdom had an

1

immediate and positive impact on services for mentally ill people. Responsibility for mental hospitals was transferred from local councils to the newly formed Northern Ireland Hospitals Authority and a highly innovative law [Mental Health Act (NI) 1948] was passed. The question is asked – why did this specific mix of policies emerge at this time? In Chapter Four, the consequences of post-war administrative and financial policies are explored. Mental hospital services, now integrated into a general hospital framework, were improved and expanded in line with standards being set in Britain. Difficulties in the operation of the new health service system were also beginning to emerge and some questioned the wisdom of importing British health policies to Northern Ireland.

Chapter Five is concerned with the impact of the outbreak of political violence (in 1969 and the years which followed) on the mental health of the people of Northern Ireland. Studies carried out by psychiatrists are examined to assess the impact of the 'troubles' on individuals. Administrative reports of the time are examined also to see if the violence had a significant effect on mental health policy or service delivery. In Chapter Six, the effect of Direct Rule on social policy, including mental health policy, is considered. The most striking trend is one of increasing convergence between Britain and Northern Ireland. As one example of the convergence in policies, the latest piece of mental health legislation [Mental Health (NI) Order 1986] is examined in terms of the influences on its formulation and implementation. In the final chapter, the impact of changes in mental health policy on the lives of six people, three men and three women, is examined. All of these people were diagnosed as having a serious mental illness involving them in psychiatric treatment both in hospital and in the community over a period of thirty years. Each story reveals complex mental health issues which can be understood only within the particular cultural context of Northern Ireland and confirms the need for policics tailored to the needs of its people.

The research for this study has been carried out against the background of literature on social policy development in Northern Ireland, histories of psychiatry in Britain and the United States, theoretical material defining mental illness, and general literature on policy analysis. A brief look at some of the mental health literature will help set the context for the Northern Ireland study.

Historical perspectives on mental health

The past thirty years have witnessed the publication of histories of mental health service development with almost because many different perspectives as there are authors. Categorization of the perspectives is extremely difficult as many of the writers see themselves as unique representatives of their own viewpoint. However, there are two distinct trends in these writings. One is the 'orthodox' approach, which is usually a 'top down' account based on official sources. It often presents changes in mental health services in terms of linear progress towards a modern and 'good' system of care and treatment for mental illness. The other presents an interpretation of developments in the light of current academic debates on the distribution of power in society. The latter are usually grouped together as 'revisionist' histories, in spite of the fact that many of the revisionist writers have little in common except their view of public mental health care systems as methods of maintaining boundaries between the sane and the insane and of creating the social construct 'mental disorder'. These trends are apparent in the literature on both the USA and Britain although the contexts (both legal and administrative) are completely different.

'Orthodox' histories

Gerald Grob (1973, 1983) is the best current American example of a historical approach based on a model of linear progress. Grob is an evolutionist who is sympathetic to modern psychiatric practice. In his study of the decline of the asylum within American psychiatry, Grob (1983) sees the gradual abandonment of the asylum as a positive step, although he argues that American society has not yet developed a coherent policy which provides 'decent and humane' care for mentally ill people. A similar approach to that of Grob is reflected in the two major histories of psychiatry, published in the 1960s, Hunter and Macalpine (1963) and Alexander and Selesnick (1966), who saw the development of psychiatry as 'a central part of the evolution of civilization itself'. (Ibid. p. 21)

Earlier examples of 'orthodox' histories which are not evolutionary in approach include the work of Albert Deutsch (1937) and Kathleen Jones (1953 and 1960). Written before the sociological debates of the 1960s, Deutsch and Jones offer accounts of policy developments in their legal and historical contexts. Jones has been criticized for being 'constrained by the medical model' (Skultans 1979, p. 3) and for being 'Whiggish' in her approach. [For discussion see Berrios and Freeman (ed) 1991] However, it is clear from her later work especially that a rigorous examination of institutions, professions and other powerful interests is an essential part of her approach, an examination which includes a critical evaluation of the contribution of the medical profession to mental health policy. (Jones 1972 and 1988; Jones and Fowles 1984)

In contrast to histories based on a model of linear progress, revisionist writers interpret all developments in treatment for mental disorder in terms of the distribution of power or of economic resources in modern sociey. The influence of the French political philosopher, Michel Foucault, and of the American sociologist Erving Goffman is evident in most of these writings. Foucault writes powerfully on a 'Great Confinement' which began with the setting up of the Hôpital Général in Paris in 1656 and which spread throughout Europe. For him the asylum was an 'instrument of moral uniformity and of social denunciation.' (Foucault 1965, p. 259) Developments in treatment have not altered the inequality of power which exists in the doctor-patient relationship. 'There remains, beyond the empty forms of positivist thought, only a single concrete reality: the doctor-patient couple in which all alienations are summarized, linked and loosened.' (Foucault 1965, p. 277) Foucault has been challenged on the empirical accuracy of his work. (Bynum et al 1985b, p. 2) but his influence continues in spite of his critics.

Erving Goffman (1961, 1971) was (and indeed still is) the other major influence on academic studies of institutional treatment for mental disorder. For Goffman, as for other deviance theorists, mental hospitals were means by which society conferred and reinforced the label 'mental disorder' on certain people whose behaviour did not fit the norm. His analysis of the interaction of staff and patients at St Elizabeth's Mental Hospital in Washington, demonstrated graphically the ways in which the institution built up and reinforced the patient role, thus preserving rather than curing the illness. By the 1960s, when Goffman was writing, many mental hospitals in the United States still retained characteristics of the 'total institution' (Goffman 1961, p. xiii) but in the United Kingdom this was changing rapidly as interaction between the 'hospital world' and the 'outside world' increased. Goffman's major contribution to the debate was to question the official view of what went on in hospitals. This questioning encompassed aspects of patient life hitherto taken for granted. Was adaptation to the role of patient healthy or pathological? Did activities such as the annual Sports Day, the hospital magazine and the Christmas concert help consolidate the patient identity thus maintaining the segregative effect of the hospital environment? How could 'real' mental illness be distinguished from the patient role performance?

This last question raises the issue of the reality of mental illness, an issue about which the American psychiatrist Thomas Szasz has written prolifically. Szasz has been questioning the existence of mental illness since the publication of his first book *The Myth of Mental Illness* in 1961. An advocate of 'contractual psychotherapy' he sees the compulsory confinement and treatment of a person in a mental hospital as representing one man's oppressive control over another. He parallels the labelling of a person as mentally ill with that of labelling a witch during the seventeenth century, and the acceptance of psychiatric definitions of mental illness with the acceptance of a religious belief. He sees the history of psychiatry as 'largely an account of changing fashions in the theory and practice of psychiatric violence, cast in the self approbating idioms of medical diagnosis and treatment'. (Szasz 1970, p. 278) Szasz however, does not reject the medical model. The psychiatrist, without any trace of moral superiority, can engage people in therapy if they are rich enough and motivated enough to seek help with what he terms 'problems of living'. Unlike many other 'revisionists' Szasz is a right-wing libertarian whose chief aim is to oppose publicly organized mental health systems whether these are hospital or community based. Szasz has been criticized by a number of authors including Jones and Fowles (1984, p. 67), and Clare (1977) because of the internal inconsistencies in his arguments. However, in spite of the fact that he is often illogical and frequently contradicts himself, Szasz has been influential in articulating a number of valuable questions : Who defines mental illness? Are psychiatric services instruments of man's oppression of man? Has society given to psychiatry the role it used to give to religion?

The influence of Foucault, Goffman and Szasz can be seen in the work of historians such as Rothman (1971 and 1980), writing in the United States, and Finnane (1981) and Malcolm (1989) writing in Ireland. In his two major histories of the development of different kinds of institutional treatment for orphans, offenders and mentally ill people, Rothman maintains his basic stance as a deviance theorist with a focus on the institution as the chief instrument of social control. Rothman has been criticized for being theoretically too narrow (failing to take social and economic factors into account) and for seeing America as different from other parts of the world when in fact similar patterns of service development were evident in Britain and other parts of Europe.

Andrew Scull is one of Rothman's most articulate critics. His own work offers a Marxist interpretation of the development of treatment for mental disorder in England since the eighteenth century. (Scull 1984 and 1989) For him the demise of the asylum in the twentieth century has to be interpreted in the same way as its emergence in the nineteenth century – as a response to the changing needs of capitalism. With the coming of the 'welfare state' segregative modes of social control became too costly and difficult to justify. (Scull 1977, p. 135) In common with Rothman, he sees mental hospital treatment as one form of the social control of deviant elements in society. He goes further than Rothman in interpreting both the development of the asylum system in the nineteenth century and the

5

policy of 'decarcerceration' in the twentieth century as caused by developments in capitalism.

Scull describes his own work as an attempt to 'develop an historically informed, macro-sociological perspective on the interrelationships between deviance, control structures and the wider social systems of which they are a part.' (Scull 1985, p. 1)] Scull continues to examine psychiatric treatment in these terms. He writes of the 'reconceptualisation of a variety of social problems as medical conditions in need of treatment' and sees this process as part of the psychiatric professions' decision to move their focus away from the 'dismal, despised and depressing institutional sector'. (Scull 1991, p. 165) Psychiatry, due to technological and pharmacological advances, can offer treatments which are adaptable to a number of settings. These new treatment techniques are, according to Scull, no less controlling than the asylums of the last century.

Other revisionist theorists include two feminist writers Skultans (1979) and Showalter (1987). The relationship between the cultural definition of femininity and the illness which emerged is particularly well documented by Showalter in relation to Victorian England. Men have always been dominant among the 'definers' and 'treatment givers' and women among the patients. Current research on women and mental health has focused on almost every aspect of a woman's life, in search of an explanation for the higher rate of reported mental illness in women. [Pilowski et al. (eds) 1991] Marriage continues to be a protective factor in mens' lives and a risk factor in womens' lives. (Paykel 1991, p. 25; Bebbington et al 1991) Child care also continues to impose extra stress on women as do the new community care policies which makes demands on women to expand their role as 'informal carers'. (Morris et al. 1991)

A review of British and American literature on mental health policy cannot ignore the legal revisionists although only one historical work from this perspective has been published – that of Clive Unsworth (1987). Unsworth is influenced by Kittrie (1971) and Gostin (1975) the two major American writers in this field. Both emphasize the need for the law to protect the individual citizen from any form of unecessary intervention in his or her life even if this was seen as 'treatment' or 'therapy'. In Kittrie's own words : 'Man's innate right to remain free of excessive forms of human modification shall be inviolable'. (Kittrie 1971, p. 402)

The editors of the recent history of the Royal College of Psychiatrists view revisionist writings with scepticism, pointing out that they 'ignore the fact that medicine's role in society is a mainly instrumental one' and that psychiatry has the particularly unpopular task of taking charge of those whose behaviour breaks society's basic rules'. [Berrios and Freeman (eds) 1991, p. xii] However, any student of mental health service

6

development must take into account the issues raised by legal, medical and sociological revisionists in order to understand the complex decisions made at different stages of this development.

Irish historical accounts

The influence of revisionist historical writing is evident in the three recent histories of mental health services in Ireland, although both Robins (1986) and Malcolm (1989) see changes in mental health services in terms of progress. The work of Finnane, an Australian historian, is more like a revisionist account. He examines the political and social factors in nineteenth century Ireland which led to the establishment of a system of public asylums. (Finnane 1981) Finnane's research is particularly relevant to the study of mental health policies in Northern Ireland, as it provides an excellent analysis of Irish lunacy provision at the beginning of the twentieth century.

The other two histories of mental health services in Ireland, Robins (1986) and Malcolm (1989), present a wealth of material on the social and economic context of these services. Robins (1986) traces beliefs about the treatment of madness from the pre-christian era, through the Brehon laws and monastic provision, to the era of confinement and the growth of the asylum system. He makes no attempt to offer a structural analysis of developments in the care of the insane but shows how each era inherits the structure of a previous age. Robins is a journalist of great skill. His work is easy to read but offers a fairly superficial account of the history of the treatment of mental disorder in Ireland.

Elizabeth Malcolm, an Australian historian, documents the history of Ireland's largest private asylum, St. Patricks Hospital, Dublin – founded by Dean Jonathan Swift in 1746. (Malcolm 1989) Her study makes a major contribution to the historical understanding of institutional care for mental disorder. Though influenced by Foucault, Malcolm dissociates herself from his main assumptions. She accepts 'the reality of psychotic and neurotic illness and the need for psychiatric treatment' but, as a historian, is interested in how 'familial, social and even political and economic factors have shaped mental illness'. (Malcolm 1989, p. ix) Some of her material on the factors which led to the committal of women to St Patrick's during the nineteenth century are particularly fascinating to those interested in the link between cultural definitions of feminity and confinement to an asylum. In this it echoes the work of Showalter (1987). Malcolm's work is relevant to the study of mental health services in Northern Ireland, as it provides valuable material on attitudes to treatment and care of the mentally ill in the Republic of Ireland during the twentieth century. However, there are gaps in Malcolm's work which

7

limit its usefulness in relation to the current research. For example, Malcolm at no point dicusses the legal framework within which St Patrick's operated, not does she analyse its role within the context of public provision.

Notwithstanding the limitations of these historical accounts as comparative material, the publication during the 1980s of three Irish studies has highlighted the lack of historical research in relation to mental health in Northern Ireland. The present study is offered in the hope that it will be the first of many. It will focus primarily on mental health policy formation and implementation, avoiding assumptions of linear progress and avoiding also one-dimensional ideological explanations from the 'far left' or the 'far right'.

The methodology used for this study was that of historical research. This included the use of official documents of Ministries and Departments concerned with mental health services, Parliamentary and Assembly Debates, and reports of mental hospitals, the Northern Ireland Hospitals Authority and of voluntary organizations such as the Northern Ireland Association for Mental Health. Documentary evidence has been supplemented by interviews with people involved in the formation and implementation of policies, by a study of case records from mental hospitals, by visits to hostels and day centres and by informal interviews with a number of patients.

1 New politics, old problems – 1921

The government of Northern Ireland was established in 1921 as a temporary measure. The size of what became known as 'the Province', its financial dependence on Great Britain, and its anomalous position within Ireland made its position extremely unstable. Its people were devastated by the Great Famine of the 1840s, diminished by the tide of emigration which followed, and exhausted by the bitterness which surrounded the political struggles of the late nineteenth and early twentieth centuries. It inherited workhouses – relics of the Poor Law – and district asylums, full of the casualties of the wider society. These were the people who had not died of starvation or political violence, who were not 'able' enough to emigrate, and who had no family members willing to support them.

The six district asylums were part of a network of 23 dotted around Ireland, a network which resulted from two waves of enthusiastic institution building, the first begun in the 1820s and the second in the 1860s. By 1921 asylum provision was an underfunded, overcrowded system of care based on numerous lunacy acts, the earliest dating from 1821. The laws reflected the history of care and confinement of lunatics in Ireland from the early nineteenth century. All were difficult to understand and complex to administer. The need for legislative reform was one of the most urgent problems inherent in the system of lunacy provision. However, lunacy reform was far from being a burning issue in a country where the fight for independence from England had been the main concern for many decades. Consequently, there had been no lunacy reform movement in Ireland and no equivalent of the English Lunacy Act 1890 (53 & 54 Vict. c. 5).

For local councils, which held both financial and administrative responsibility for the asylums, the most pressing problem was financial. Though central funding of patients on a per capita basis had been introduced in 1875 [PRO(NI) CAB 9B/176/1], this funding had been eroded in real terms after 1898 due to the dwindling resources of the Irish tax reserve, and to the rapid increase in the cost of living after the outbreak of war in 1914. (Finnane 1981, p. 57: Malcolm 1989, p. 239) These problems were carried over into the new political and administrative structure of Northern Ireland in 1921. The impact of legal complexity and inadequate funding on mental health policy formation and service delivery on Northern Ireland was far reaching. It accounted for the total lack of development in mental health services between 1921 and 1948. To understand this impact we look first at the political situation in Northern Ireland as it emerged in 1921.

The birth of a new political order

Northern Ireland came into existence with a Parliament established on the Westminster model, devolved from it but subordinate to it. The new political unit consisted of six of the nine counties which form the province of Ulster – Antrim, Down, Armagh, Fermanagh, Londonderry and Tyrone. The decisions on boundaries were based on religious and political rather than on economic considerations and were intended as temporary measures pending an all Ireland settlement. (Buckland 1981, p. 20; Wilson 1989, p. 56) The settlement envisaged by the British government did not materialize and, as a result, from 1921 onwards Northern Ireland developed independently from the rest of Ireland both administratively and politically. The political settlement served only to mask the existence of different political aspirations within the population of Northern Ireland. It continued to be a divided society with two distinct communities each drawing its identity from its religious affiliation. (For further discussion see Arthur 1980, Ch. 3; Rose 1971, Ch. XV) These divisions permeated every layer of social interaction and were manifested in many different ways including the eruption of political violence at irregular intervals and the frequent allegations of discriminatory practice levelled at local government officials.

The impact of the political and administrative changes on specific aspects of life are difficult to reconstruct. Asylum records present us only with snippets of information on what was really happening. For example, in the minutes of the Management Committee of the Belfast Asylum the transfer of administrative responsibility from Dublin to Belfast was acknowledged, and a motion passed that 'the gratitude of the committee for help received be conveyed to officials in Dublin.' [PRO(NI) HOS 28/1/1/14] In Downpatrick, the Management Committee of the asylum passed a resolution to welcome the King and Queen to the opening of

Parliament and merely noted the administrative changeover to the Ministry of Home Affairs in Belfast. [PRO(NI) HOS 14/1/2/2]

The only inkling of trouble which can be gleaned from these minutes came when staff of both asylums were asked to sign a declaration of allegiance to the British monarchy (under Section 5(2) of the Local Government Act (NI) 1920. In each asylum, the Catholic chaplain refused to sign the declaration. When informed that their contracts would be terminated because of this refusal, they responded differently. The chaplain in Downpatrick, on the advice of his bishop, refused to sign and the position was left vacant at great inconvenience to staff and patients. The chaplain in Belfast conformed to the law and stayed in his job. [PRO(NI) HOS 28/1/1/14 and HOS 14/1/2/3] Incidents such as those merely give us hints of the kinds of disruptions which must have occurred during this period of transition. Due to the way in which electoral ward boundaries had been drawn (ensuring a majority of Protestant seats), the majority of local councils with responsibility for district asylums were committed to supporting the Unionist state. (See Wilson 1989, p. 69) However, there must have been some members of staff who, like the chaplains, did not wish to sign a declaration of allegiance. If they existed they did not make any formal protest.

Parliamentary and administrative upheaval

Central control over this divided society was held by the Northern Ireland Parliament which, like the Westminster Parliament, was bi-cameral. Parliamentary procedure was similar to that in Westminster. There was, however one major difference between the two Parliaments. The powers exercised by the Northern Ireland Parliament were extremely limited because of its subordinate position within the United Kingdom. The impact of this subordinate position was felt in all aspects of government policy in Northern Ireland and some of the major difficulties experienced within the mental health services were due directly to the limitations imposed by it.

The legal basis of Parliamentary power, established in the Government of Ireland Act 1920, failed to anticipate the difficulties which would be encountered by a six-counties administration. (Buckland 1981, pp. 21-24) There were several areas in which the new Parliament had no power and the way in which its financial affairs were arranged left Northern Ireland with very little opportunity for independent action. It had no control over its revenue and little over its expenditure. (See Lawrence 1965, p. 21) Original estimates of both revenue and expenditure for Northern Ireland proved inaccurate during the early 1920s. Revenue was lower and expenditure higher than anticipated. This led to a situation described by Harkness (1983, p. 5) as 'two decades of frustration, irritation and hand to mouth existence.' The British government was not in favour of subsidising Northern Ireland, a fact which was evident in Cabinet papers of the time. 'It is imperative that British aid be transient only, and that within a reasonable time an autonomous Ireland must be able to rely on her own resources.' [Paper on finance by Sir Ernest Clarke in PRO(NI) D 1022/2/22]

Of the seven departments created in 1921 for the administration of Northern Ireland two were influential in relation to mental health services. The Ministry for Home Affairs held overall responsibility for health care but decisions on policies which involved expenditure were in the hands of the Ministry of Finance. The two Ministers, Sir R. Dawson Bates (Home Affairs) and Hugh Pollock (Finance), represented different approaches to government policy in Northern Ireland. Dawson Bates, together with Sir J. Craig (Prime Minister), favoured an approach characterized by high consumption of public funds and the achievement of parity with Britain in all matters related to public and social services. (Bew, Gibbon and Patterson 1979) Pollock, supported by Sir Wilfred Spender (Secretary to the Minister of Finance and head of the Northern Ireland Civil Service) and backed by the Westminster Treasury, opposed the automatic extension of social reforms to Northern Ireland and favoured economic stringency. [PRO(NI) D 1022/2/22] It was this view which shaped health expenditure during the 1920s and 1930s.

Before 1921, administrative responsibility for mental health services throughout Ireland had been held by the Lunacy Inspectorate for Ireland, based in Dublin. This Inspectorate, established in the mid nineteenth century, had lost a great deal of its power by the beginning of the twentieth century. This was due to two factors – the loss of control by central government agencies in Dublin (agencies which represented British rule in Ireland) due to the pre-dominance of the national question at the end of the century, and the establishment in 1898 of local councils. [Local Government (Ireland) Act: 61 & 62 Vict. c. 37] By the 1920s, local councils were exercising almost complete control over district asylums with the Lunacy Inspectorate playing only a monitoring role. In 1921 the Lunacy Inspectorate split as administratvie responsibility for lunacy services in Northern Ireland moved to Belfast. The new Inspectorate functioned from within the Ministry of Home Affairs. The immediate effects (on mental health policy) of the transfer of political and administrative power were the freezing of the central government grant to asylums at the pre-1921 level [PRO(NI) CAB 9B/176/1] and the further delay of any preparation for changes in the law. In a Province torn by political strife and bowed down by economic depression, services for mentally ill people rated very low on the priority list.

To understand later changes we look first at the services as they existed in 1921.

Mental health services in 1921

One of the major difficulties in writing about this period stems from changing social perceptions of what had been defined as lunacy in the nineteenth century. Existing lunacy laws and services were based on definitions which began to lose credibility in the early years of the twentieth century. Asylums had been built in Ireland to control the problem of the insane confined in prisons and those 'wandering at large'. [HMSO(Irl) 1817] The philosophy of moral management, in vogue in the early part of the century, was quickly replaced by that of medical treatment. In 1835, Dr Robert Stuart (of Belfast Asylum) was appointed as the first medical superintendent in a district asylum in Ireland and in 1862 a medical qualification became a prerequisite for the post of asylum manager. (Finnane 1981, p. 47; Williamson 1970, p. 290) At that time the medical profession had little to offer in terms of treatment for mental illness, but the expansion of district asylums proved fertile ground for the emergence of psychiatry as a new specialism within medicine.

By the early twentieth century, it was accepted by the public that asylums existed not only to protect society but also to provide medical treatment. The negative effect of this change in public perception was the removal of the lunacy question from the arena of public debate and 'the decline of lay interest and involvement' (Finnane 1981, p. 47) This loss of interest was compounded by the existence of other major concerns in Ireland in the late nineteenth and early twentieth century where the struggle for national independence dominated the political agenda. It was therefore politically expedient to accept the emerging definition of lunacy as illness, and leave it to the medical profession and local government officials to administer services peripheral to the main concerns of the country.

However, the language used in official reports show that there was still confusion concerning mental disorder and its treatment. Concepts of 'lunacy' and 'insanity' were still widely used although interspersed with concepts of 'illness' and 'treatment'. Examples of this mixture of old and new rhetoric are to be found in the *First Report of the Inspectors of Lunacy (NI)* for 1921 and 1922.

> We have so far dealt with the number of the insane in institutions . . . but as already stated this does not include all the insane, as a number reside in their own homes or with relatives or are wandering at large . . . . In 1922 three patients escaped and were not retaken . . . . The mentally affected inmates in all the workhouses

visited during the last two years bore the appearance of being well cared for. [HMSO(NI) 1924, pp. 8-13]

Some of this language echoed that used in prison reports and some that of health reports. However, though the language of official documents was still often that of 'control', policies were changing. The asylum system, which at the beginning of the nineteenth century had as its intended outcome the control of vagrancy, could no longer be said to have overt social control functions. Due to the serious political divisions within Irish society, the British government was intensely concerned with maintaining law and order. However, lunatics were no longer re-garded as posing a serious threat to public order and political interest and government intervention in lunacy policies were minimal in the late nineteenth and early twentieth centuries.

The institutions

In 1921 services for people with a mental disorder were dominated by the six district asylums at Armagh, Antrim, Belfast, Derry, Omagh and Downpatrick. There was only one private asylum – the Quaker Retreat at Armagh, which together with a small number of nursing homes, offered private care for single certified patients. These services were supplemented by workhouses which offered care to elderly patients suffering from senile dementia and to adults and children with a mental handicap. In addition, criminals deemed insane by the courts were sent to the Central Criminal Lunatic Asylum (established 1845) in Dundrum, Dublin. Responsibility for administering the district asylums and work-houses lay with the six county and two county borough councils (estab-lished in 1898) and overall responsibility for policy making and implementation lay with the office of the Inspectors of Lunatics within the Department of Home Affairs. The following extract from the first report of the Inspectors of Lunatics in Northern Ireland summarizes the services in 1921 (See Figure 1.1).

District asylums : As can be seen from the summary of patient numbers, 4,277 people (or 3.4 per 1,000 of the population) were receiving institu-tional care in different settings in 1921. The majority of these – 93 per cent were in asylums. The other seven per cent were in workhouses, private asylums or in the Central Criminal Lunatic Asylum, Dublin. Though not as high as the national figure, patient numbers in Northern Ireland were following the same upward trend as in other parts of Ireland. (See Appendix 1) The number of asylum patients had been increasing steadily throughout Ireland during the late nineteenth and early twentieth centuries both in real terms and as a proportion of the

FIRST REPORT

OF THE

INSPECTORS OF LUNATICS

ON THE

District and Private Lunatic Asylums

IN NORTHERN IRELAND.

To THE RIGHT HONOURABLE SIR RICHARD DAWSON BATES,
Minister of Home Affairs for Northern Ireland.

MINISTRY OF HOME AFFAIRS,
OCEAN BUILDINGS,
DONEGALL SQUARE EAST.
BELFAST,
5th January, 1924.

SIR,

We have the honour to submit to you, for presentation to His Grace the Governor of Northern Ireland, our Report on the condition and management of Lunatics and Lunatic Asylums in Northern Ireland for the period from 1st December, 1921, to 31st December, 1922, including Northern Ireland cases located in the Central Criminal Lunatic Asylum at Dundrum, Co. Dublin.

The following Summary shows the number and distribution of the insane under official cognizance on the 31st December, 1922, as compared with the number and distribution on 31st December, 1920 and 1921 :—

—	On 31st December, 1920.			On 31st December, 1921.			On 31st December, 1922.		
	Males.	Fe-males.	Total.	Males.	Fe-males.	Total.	Males.	Fe-males.	Total.
In District Asylums	2 107	1,876	3,983	2,089	1,866	3,955	2,080	1,885	3,965
Northern Ireland cases located in Central Criminal Lunatic Asylum, Dundrum, County Dublin	18	5	23	24	5	29	22	6	28
In The Private Asylum	10	29	39	8	30	38	5	33	38
In Workhouses	83	108	191	92	109	201	100	122	222
Chancery Patients and *Single Patients in Unlicensed Houses	11	13	24	†10	†14	†24	9	15	24
Totals	2,229	2,031	4,260	2,223	2,024	4,247	2,216	2,061	4,277

* i.e., individual cases, it being illegal to detain more than one insane person in any unlicensed house. (5 & 6 Vic. c. 123, sec. 3).

† These numbers are approximate, as, owing to the destruction of documents in Dublin, the exact figures could not be obtained.

The foregoing numbers do not include the insane wandering at large or those residing in private dwellings, with the exception of such cases as are under the care of the Lord Chief Justice, i.e., Chancery patients.

Figure 1.1   Extract from first report of Inspectors of Lunatics (NI) 1921

Source: *HMSO (NI) 1924*

population. In 1900, for example, the number of patients resident in district asylums in Ireland (including Northern Ireland) was 3.8 per 1,000. By 1910 this figure had reached 4.7 and by 1920 it was 5.5 per 1,000. [HMSO(Irl) 1921; Finnane 1981, p. 233]

In contrast to the workhouse system, which by the early twentieth century was beginning to decline, asylums continued to occupy a significant position in Irish life. (Finnane 1981, pp. 33 & 223; Burke 1987) This was true not only because of the treatment they offered to people suffering from a mental disorder but also because of their social and economic importance. District asylums were important employers in areas which often had no other major industry as well as being important consumers of local goods and services. There were six of these asylums in Northern Ireland. The oldest – Armagh Asylum – had been built in 1825 and was in fact the first district asylum in Ireland. The newest, Antrim Asylum, had been built in 1899 to cope with the increased demand for beds in the greater Belfast area. By 1921 the Belfast Asylum had been moved to a new site outside of the city and in Derry an additional hospital had been built at Gransha. [HMSO(NI) 1924] The other four asylums remained virtually unaltered except for some minor extensions and improvements.

When asylums were first built in Ireland in the early nineteenth century, accommodation was planned for some 100 patients in each. Very soon the numbers seeking admission far outstripped beds available. From his detailed study of asylum admissions in the late nineteenth century, Finnane (1981, p. 136) concluded that the increase in demand was related to changing farming practices, to emigration, and to a decline in marriage, though none of these factors in themselves can totally explain the ease with which people were committed to the asylum. As the numbers seeking admission increased during the century, more accommodation was provided. In spite of this effort, by 1921 buildings were severely overcrowded and conditions grossly inadequate. In Belfast plans for expansion were already underway.

> In this asylum also there is considerable overcrowding, but the Committee of Management are fully alive to the necessity for remedying this state of affairs, and have decided on a scheme of building to be spread over a term of years, in order to complete and extend the original plan of the Villa colony Asylum at Purdysburn. [HMSO(NI) 1924, p. 11]

Table 1.1 shows the overall trend in patient numbers in the six district asylums in Northern Ireland since their establishment.

Asylums built in the 1820s had a capacity of approximately one hundred beds in each as the early lunacy reformers had been optimistic that the treatment offered within asylums would lead to a fairly rapid turn-

Table 1.1
Patient population in district asylums 1921

Name of asylum	Year opened	Original bed number	Patients 1921 (daily average)
Antrim	1899	400	513
Armagh	1825	104	510
Belfast	1829	104	985
Downpatrick	1869	300	701
Derry	1829	104	491
Omagh	1853	300	773

Sources: Finnane 1981; HMSO(NI) 1924

over in the patient population. However, this did not happen and during the second wave of asylum building in the 1860s, the average capacity had increased to 300 beds. The most rapid increase in patients occurred after 1875 when there was a shift in financing from local taxation to a 'grant in aid of local taxation'. Between 1870 and 1914 the population of district asylums throughout Ireland trebled from approximately 7,000 to 21,000. (Finnane 1981, p. 53; Raftery 1985, p. 287) During the early part of this period – from 1875 to 1898 (the year in which local councils were established), asylum administrators had ensured that full use was made of the per capita grant. Though the original intention was that the grant would correspond to half of the actual cost per patient (up to a maximum of four shillings), in most instances the full amount was paid. By the middle of the 1890s the Treasury grant covered over 50 per cent of asylum costs with some such as Omagh District Asylum, receiving as much as 65 per cent of its total costs. [Finnane 1981, p. 58; PRO(NI) CAB 9B/176/1]

After 1898 the situation changed. The Local Government (Ireland) Act 1898 (s. 58) provided for the continuance of the principle introduced in 1875. The only difference was that in future the grant would be paid from the newly created Local Taxation (Ireland) Account, subject to there being enough funds in the account. Because part of the income for this account was derived from liquor licenses, the actual amount of money in the Taxation Account fluctuated. Unfortunately, its funds decreased during the early twentieth century as did also the allocation for asylums. By 1921, therefore, the financial burden was firmly placed on local councils with the government capitation grant constituting only 13 per cent of total income to the six district asylums. [HMSO(NI) 1924, p. 40]

Any hope that councils may have had for a speedy solution to this problem were soon dispelled. In 1921 the Local Taxation (Ireland) Account was abolished. In 1923 the Local Government Act provided for the payment of a fixed grant equivalent to the average payment from this account for the three years preceding 1921. This amounted to a total of £37,079 per year – an amount which was to be divided proportionately between the six asylums. [PRO(NI) CAB 9B/176/1] This was clearly inadequate but was intended as a temporary measure.

However, it soon became clear that there was little hope for an increase in central funding as Northern Ireland struggled to avoid bankrupcy. The 1920s saw a decline in world demand for the products of the three major industries in the Province – linen, ship-building and agriculture. (Johnson 1985, p. 188) Furthermore, a subvention from the Westminster Treasury was out of the question because of its own financial difficulties in the aftermath of the war. Fortunately for local councils, there had been a temporary drop in patient numbers during the 1914-18 war with the result that the average number of patients resident in the asylums remained static between 1919 and 1924.

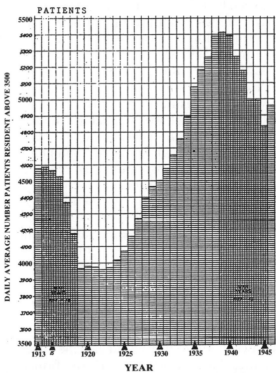

Figure 1.2 Daily average of patients resident in district asylums 1913-46

Source: *HMSO (NI) 1948a, p.56*

The lull caused by the decrease in patient numbers gave the councils a temporary breathing space. However, it did not alter the situation in any significant way and the combination of inadequate funding and lack of public interest led to a period of utter stagnation in the development of a better environment for the care of patients in the six district asylums in Northern Ireland. This period lasted for twenty seven years – from 1921 to 1948.

However, even during this period of stagnation, a number of patients did seem to benefit from asylum care. The Casebooks (containing medical records) for the Downpatrick Asylum record a number of successful discharges. Some of these patients, admitted because of their bizarre or depressed behaviour, improved without any medical intervention, having seen a doctor only once during their stay in the asylum. The main factor determining their discharge seems to have been the willingness of a family member to take them home. For the majority of patients their fate was to remain in the asylum until they died. It is clear from case records that in the midst of political trouble and strife, life continued as normal within the asylum. Patients were admitted and cared for in a way which required only an adequate diet, some exercise and an occasional visit by a doctor. When behaviour improved the patient was discharged if members of the family were willing to take responsibility. If not the patient was destined to become part of the long stay population open to all of the health risks of a closed institution with poor medical and sanitary facilities. (Downpatrick Asylum Casebooks 1920-1930).

The level of care being offered was determined largely by the quality of staffing at the time. By the 1920s, psychiatry was well established as a specialty within medicine in England. In Ireland, though there were only a small number of doctors involved in asylum care, they were the most powerful group within the system, due largely to the influence of Doctors Francis White and John Nugent, the first Inspectors of Lunacy in Ireland. (Finnane 1981, p. 42) From an initial position (during the mid nineteenth century) of total control over matters such as staffing and finance within the asylum, the role of the Resident Medical Superintendent (RMS) had diminished by the 1920s. The relationship between him (it was never a woman) and the hospital management committee was sometimes difficult because of an overlap in functions. Conflicts often arose in relation to decisions involving extra expenditure. For example in the early 1920s, the management committee at Belfast District Asylum was extremely irate that the Resident Medical Superintendent had decided to introduce (without approval) new conditions of work (a 56 hour week) for nursing staff – a change which would necessitate the employment of additional nurses. [PRO(NI) HOS 28/1/1/13] Medical staff, though at the top of the asylum hierarchy, had little power to improve services because of the financial stranglehold within which they operated.

The largest group of staff in asylums were the attendants, an unqualified group of men and women who were often hired because of their physical strength rather than their education or understanding of mental disorder. The majority of these attendants were members of the Irish Asylum Workers Union which was formed when the Irish Branch of the British Asylum Workers Association split off from the main body in 1917. [HMSO(Irl) 1921, p. xiv; Robins 1986, p. 183] In an effort to improve salaries and other conditions of service the Union immediately became involved in negotiations with local councils. After a series of bitter strikes, supported in some asylums by patients, new salary scales and a 56 hour working week were introduced in most asylums in 1920. [Robins 1986, pp. 183-86; Malcolm 1989, p. 240; PRO(NI) HOS 14/1/2/2]

Unfortunately, during the years immediately following the partition of Ireland, workers in Northern Ireland lost their bargaining power because the unions to which they belonged no longer operated in the same social and political milieu. Though many continued to be members of the Irish Asylum Workers Union, the Union itself was not in a position to exert pressure on central or local government in Northern Ireland. In effect, the attendants in Northern Ireland had lost their collective bargaining power and had to rely on the 'goodwill' of local councils and the Resident Medical Superintendent of the asylum in which they worked. This became evident in 1922 when the advantages gained in 1920 were lost as local councils reduced the salaries of all staff in the asylums because of a drop in the cost of living during the post-war period. [PRO(NI) HOS 28/1/1/14]

The insane in workhouses In 1921 there were twenty five workhouses in Northern Ireland each with an infirmary attached to it. In 1929, efforts to dissociate hospital treatment from poor relief resulted in the closure of two workhouses and the upgrading to district hospitals of six workhouse infirmaries. Plans to close more workhouses and to upgrade others involved serious consideration of the resident population, including the 201 workhouse patients who appeared in the lunacy statistics in 1921. (See Figure 1.1) These were people who had been transferred there from district asylums, under the Lunatics Asylums (Ireland) Act 1875 (38 & 39 Vict. c. 67) This Act prescribed that:

> The guardians of any poor law union in Ireland may receive into the workhouse of such union any chronic lunatic not being dangerous, who may have been received into a district lunatic asylum, and selected by the resident medical superintendent thereof and certified by him to be fit and proper so to be removed . . . and thereupon

every such lunatic so long as he shall remain in such workhouse, shall continue a patient on the books of the asylum ... and any expense incurred by the board of governors in respect of such lunatic in such workhouse shall be deemed part of the expenses of such district lunatic asylum, and shall be paid by the governors out of the moneys applicable to the payment of such expenses. [Lunatic Asylims (Ireland) Act 1875, s.9]

During this period, admission to the workhouse was often used as an overflow mechanism by district asylums. Those transferred tended to be elderly people suffering from senile dementia and young patients with a mental handicap. Belfast workhouse had the highest number (75 in 1921) in this category. This was almost certainly due to the fact that the district asylum in Belfast was severely overcrowded. [HMSO(NI) 1924, pp. 16 & 46) Only two other workhouses in the Province had a significant number of patients of 'unsound mind' – Lurgan, with 44 and Armagh town, with 34. (Ibid)

The 'insane in workhouses' in 1921, though they constituted only five per cent of the total number of people institutionalized for mental disorder, were an important group of people. They were doubly stigmatized by being transferred from asylums to institutions which were regarded as the last resort of the poor. For these people there was little hope of treatment or of discharge. The expectations of the Inspectorate of Lunacy in relation to their care were low. To use a modern phrase, 'warehousing' was lauded as good care.

> The mentally affected inmates in all the Workhouses visited during the last two years bore the appearance of being well cared for. Their clothing was, upon the whole, satisfactory and their accommodation, although in some instances lacking in cheerfulness was clean and well kept .... The beds were in general of modern form, comfortable and, with trifling exceptions, in good order, but a few old fashioned straw beds were occasionally found .... The bathing arrangements were for the most part reasonably good, but the sanitation left a good deal to be desired in some instances. [HMSO(NI) 1924, p. 13]

While it could not be denied that these people were being fed, housed and clothed to some minimum standard, there is no evidence in the reports of this era that there was any real interest in their state of mind, the reasons for them being there in the first instance, or the purpose of the care being offered.

Private care Private asylums or 'registered houses' were small establishments which were registered, under the Private Lunatic Asylums

(Ireland) Act 1842, to take people who were certified as being of 'unsound mind'. Strict legal rules existed in relation to admissions and discharges and the communication of statistical information to the Inspectorate of Lunatics. The only private asylum in Northern Ireland in 1921 was the Retreat at Armagh. It had been opened by the Society of Friends in 1827, based on the principles of moral management introduced in 1796 in the first Quaker Retreat at York. Armagh was one of three Quaker Retreats in Ireland, the first of which had been opened in 1810 at Bloomfield, Co. Dublin. Residents were fully supported financially by their relatives as there was never any tradition of government funding of private care of the insane in Ireland.

In England, guardians of Poor Law Unions had used 'private madhouses' during the nineteenth century to board out difficult lunatics from workhouses (Parry-Jones 1972). In Ireland, private asylums were not used to supplement public provision and consequently many proprietors catered for small numbers and were licensed for short periods only. Though the number of patients in the Retreat during the 1920s and 1930s never exceeded 40, it continued to function until 1948 as a small but important part of the system of care for people with a mental disorder. The lack of expansion in private madhouses in Ireland was due not only to the absence of a system of boarding out insane workhouse inmates during the nineteenth century, but also to the existence of private care (for those who wished to pay for it) within district asylums. Although built for the insane poor, Irish asylums did not form part of the Poor Law administration, and were open to paying patients. The numbers were never very high – for example in 1873 there were only 166 paying patients (out of a total patient population of 9,417) in district asylums in Ireland. [HMSO(Irl) 1874, pp. 183 and 204] An examination of the records of the asylums at Belfast and Down Asylums, reveals that many of the patients who were admitted as 'paying patients' soon became 'rate aided' patients. Asylum management committees usually agreed to any reasonable offer from a relative to make a reduced payment. The patient Sarah Sargent was typical. Her father wrote to the committee of the Down District Asylum:

> Re the bill for £24 for care and maintenance of my daughter Sarah at your asylum for four years. I beg to say that as my boys who used to contribute toward her are now married, and one is in the trenches, I am unable to pay so much in future. I stated on the 12th inst. what my income is and having sold a pony, I propose to pay £12 now and £3 yearly during my lifetime. I shall forward the £12 as soon as I hear from you and the £1.10 shillings regularly half yearly. I must get a donkey instead of a pony as I cannot go on foot to town and about.

We had arrears to pay for her in the Retreat when my children ceased to pay for her, and the rebuilding of this house absorbed all my money. [PRO(NI) HOS 14/1/2/1]

The committee agreed to his proposal as it seemed reasonable in the circumstances. In many cases, however, families did not reply to the committee's request for money and the patient was transferred to the rate-aided list without further ado. The idea of promoting and expanding private care within asylums did not emerge until the early 1920s when local councillors realized that fees could be a substantial source of income. Members of the management committee of Belfast Asylum visited England to look at private asylums, and plans were drawn up for two villas for 'lower middle class' patients in addition to the existing private accommodation at Purdysburn House. The fees were different in each – at one guinea per week for the villa accommodation and three to five guineas per week for Purdysburn House. [PRO(NI) HOS 28/1/1/13, Minutes 15 Nov. 1918]

Criminal lunatics The Lunacy (Ireland) Act 1821 first made provision for two classes of criminal lunatics: persons indicted and acquitted on the grounds of insanity ; and persons found insane on indictment. After the passing of this Act both categories of prisoner were removed from prison to the local district asylum. The notion that prison was not suitable for the criminally insane was reaffirmed in 1838 by the Dangerous Lunatics (Ireland) Act (1 Vict. c. 27), which gave powers to the court to commit a criminal to prison and from there to an asylum. It also authorized the Lord Lieutenant to remove to asylums insane persons committed for trial and insane prisoners under sentence. The next development came in 1850 when the Central Criminal Asylum was opened in Dundrum, Co. Dublin, for the criminally insane who had committed a serious offence. As this was an all Ireland facility, it was used by district asylums in Ulster when then need arose. In 1921 there were 29 patients from Northern Ireland in Dundrum. An interim arrangement was made by the Ministry of Home Affairs to allow for the continued use of this facility until Northern Ireland established its own. [HMSO(NI) 1926, p. 6]

In 1929 a section of Derry prison was allocated for this purpose and renamed the Northern Ireland Criminal Lunatic Asylum. [HMSO(NI) 1930a, p. 30] By this time, there were 26 patients from Northern Ireland in Dundrum. Of these only five had not completed their sentences, so they were transferred to Derry. The others were admitted to the district asylum nearest their home. Almost all of these people had been found guilty of manslaughter or murder, but not all were viewed as violent. They merged into the district asylums in Northern Ireland as part of the ordinary patient population. Close supervision and locked doors were part of the ordinary routine of asylum life. These patients were only different from the others because they had committed a crime. The Northern Ireland Criminal Lunatic Asylum at Derry continued in operation for 15 years, after which (due to underusage) it reverted to being an ordinary prison. [HMSO(NI) 1948c]

Like the patients in asylums and workhouses, 'criminal lunatics' were almost invisible in the early years of Northern Ireland's existence. Their strange behaviour had alienated them from their families whose only option was to commit them to the care of a system which had little to offer in terms of cure or treatment. The general public had no interest in mental disorder, being more concerned with the political situation at the time. Their lack of interest was compounded by the fact that services for people with a mental disorder were based on nineteenth century laws the language of which was both frightening and stigmatizing. A closer look at these laws will perhaps help us understand the public attitude to asylums and to the patients in them.

The law and mental disorder

The legal framework within which lunacy services operated in 1921 was, like the services themselves, deeply rooted in the ideologies of the nineteenth century. There had been no equivalent in Ireland of the English Lunacy Act 1890 which rationalized and amended earlier laws governing the care and control of citizens of 'unsound mind'. As a result of this the law on mental disorder in England was reasonably clear (if highly legalistic) in 1921. (See Jones 1960 & 1972: Unsworth 1987) In contrast to this, Northern Ireland inherited a complex mix of legislation dating from 1821. Attempts to amend certain aspects of the law in the late nineteenth century had not met with any success due to the constant opposition by local interests to any measure which might increase the financial burden on the Poor Rate. (Finnane 1981, p. 103)

The underlying assumptions of this legal framework derived from society's attitude to vagrants and to the poor. Though district asylums in Ireland were not part of Poor Law administration, by the beginning of the twentieth century Poor Law attitudes were highly visible in the asylum provision and measures to ensure that nobody was an unecessary burden on the rates were built into procedures for admission and discharge. The following table outlines the main laws in operation from 1921 until the first major change took place in the form of the Mental Treatment Act (NI) 1932.

24

There were two distinct elements in this legal framework: the statutory basis for the administration and financing of asylums and the statutory basis for admissions to institutions of different types.

Table 1.2
The law and mental disorder 1921-32

A.   The Legal Basis for Asylum Administration

  - Lunacy (Ireland) Act 1821 (1 & 2 Geo. 1V, c. 33)
  - Private Lunatics Asylums (Ireland) Act 1842
    (5 & 6 Vict. c. 123)
  - Central Criminal Lunatic Asylum (Ireland) Act 1845
    (8 & 9 Vict. c. 107)
  - Lunatic Asylums (Ireland) Act 1875 (38 & 39 Vict. c. 67)
  - Local Government (Ireland) Act 1898 (61 & 62 Vict. c. 37)
  - Lunacy (Ireland) Act 1901 (1 Edw. 7, c. 17)
  - Asylum Officers Superannuation (Ireland) Act 1909
    (9 Edw. 7, c. 48)

B.   The Legal Basis for Admissions to Institutions

1   *Ordinary admissions to district asylums*
      - Local Government (Ireland) Act 1898, Sect. 9(6)

2   *Admission as a Dangerous Lunatic* to district asylums
      - Lunacy (Ireland) Act 1867, S. 10 (30 & 31 Vict. c. 118)

3   *Admission as a Criminal Lunatic*
  - By Order of the Governor of Northern Ireland
  - Army Act 1881, Sect. 91
  - Naval Enlistment Act 1884, Sect. 3
  - Poor Law Act (Scotland) 1898, Sect. 6 (61 & 62 Vict. c. 21)
  - Lunatic Asylums (Ireland) Act 1875, Sect. 12

4   *Transfer from Asylum to Workhouse*
      - Lunatic Asylums (Ireland) Act 1875, Sect. 9

5   *Admission to Private Asylums*
      - Private Lunatic Asylums (Ireland) Act 1842

Sources: *Reports of Inspectors of Lunatics (NI) 1921-26; Mental Treatment Act (NI) 1932*

The legislation did not include any precise definition of the sort of mental conditions regarded as 'lunacy', 'idiocy', 'insanity', or 'unsoundness of mind' but it was generally accepted that there was a distinction between the medical and legal definitions of insanity. Abraham (1886), in his major treatise on *Law and Practice of Lunacy in Ireland*, summarized the legal position as follows :

> The jurist views the condition of mind called lunacy or insanity with an exclusive eye to its effect upon the doings of the lunatic ... Considered in his capacity of citizen, the person alleged to be of unsound mind may, through apparent absence or disorder of intellect, create the belief among his friends and neighbours that he ought to be placed under tutelage, for safety of person and property; and it is to the judicial ascertainment of the truth on this particular that the common inquisition of office is directed. (Abraham 1886, p. 13)

Judicial certification was seen in terms of protection for the person of unsound mind against possible exploitation, or for the safety of others. Medical certification had a different function. It established that the mental disorder could be treated or contained within a publicly funded institution. (See HMSO 1957, p. 46) Table 1.3 from the *First Report of the Inspectors of Lunatics (NI)* shows the use of the laws governing admission to district asylums in 1921.

Asylum admission procedures

Though there were a number of different laws which could be used in admitting a person to a district asylum, these could be reduced to three basic methods of admission. 1) Admission as a person of unsound mind; 2) Admission as a dangerous lunatic; 3) Admission as a criminal lunatic.

Admission as a person of unsound mind This method of admission was based on the laws of the early nineteenth century which had led to the establishment of lunatic asylums for people who were both poor and insane. Early procedures involved an application to the asylum manager by the next of kin, who had to affirm the poverty of the patient and give an undertaking to remove him from the asylum when requested. This application was accompanied by a medical certificate of insanity. The decision to admit was made by the governors of the asylum. (Robins 1986, p. 143) Later on in the century, when fee-paying patients were allowed to use these institutions, it became necessary to protect these people from the possibility of improper detention. [Lunatic Asylums (Ireland) Act 1875, Sect. 16]

Table 1.3
Legal basis for admissions to district asylums 1920-21

AUTHORITY.	1920 Antrim M.	F.	Armagh M.	F.	Belfast M.	F.	Downpatrick M.	F.	Londonderry M.	F.	Omagh M.	F.	Total M.	F.	1921 Antrim M.	F.	Armagh M.	F.	Belfast M.	F.	Downpatrick M.	F.	Londonderry M.	F.	Omagh M.	F.	Total M.	F.
Admitted under Statutory Regulations made in pursuance of the Act, 61 & 62 Vic., Cap. 37, Sec. 9 (6) ..	29	36	15	22	106	110	36	51	24	29	26	28	236	276	25	26	8	18	80	116	25	40	24	31	20	41	182	272
Committed as Dangerous Lunatics under the Act, 30 & 31 Vic., Cap. 118, Sec. 10	24	22	26	17	17	3	30	12	23	18	95	51	215	123	36	13	25	20	18	5	29	26	25	21	83	42	216	127
CRIMINAL LUNATICS: Admitted by order of Lord Lieutenant ..	-	-	-	-	1	-	-	-	3	-	-	-	4	-	-	-	-	1	1	-	-	-	-	-	-	-	1	1
Committed under Army Act, 1881, Sec. 91	-	-	1	-	7	-	-	-	2	-	-	-	10	-	-	-	1	-	3	-	-	-	1	-	-	-	5	-
Committed under Naval Enlistment Act, 1884, Sec. 3	-	-	-	-	-	-	-	-	-	-	-	-	-	-	-	-	-	-	2	-	-	-	-	-	-	-	2	-
Transferred from Criminal Lunatic Asylum on expiration of sentence under Act, 38 & 39 Vic., Cap. 67, Sec.12	1	-	-	-	-	-	-	-	-	-	-	-	1	-	1	-	-	-	-	1	1	1	-	-	-	-	2	2
Admitted under Sheriff's Warrant in pursuance of Poor Law Act (Scotland), 1808, Sec. 8 ..	-	-	-	-	-	-	-	-	-	-	-	-	-	-	-	-	-	-	-	-	-	-	2	-	2	-	4	-
TOTAL ..	54	58	42	39	131	113	66	63	52	47	121	79	466	399	62	39	34	39	104	122	56	67	51	52	105	83	412	402

Source: HMSO (NI) 1924, p. 20

27

The introduction of the requirement for two medical certificates of 'unsoundness of mind' (for private patients) was aimed at preventing any abuses.

With the establishment of local councils in 1898, it became necessary to update admission procedures. The Local Government (Ireland) Act 1898, which changed the administrative framework of district asylums, made it the duty of the newly formed county councils to provide accommodation for the lunatic poor, and to manage the asylum for the county. It also gave power to the council to

> ... make regulations respecting the government and management of every lunatic asylum for their county, and the admission, detention and discharge of lunatics, and the conditions as to payment and accommodation under which private patients may be admitted into and detained in the asylum ... [Local Government (Irl) Act 1898, Sect. 9(6)]

From 1921 until 1932 the standard method of admission to district asylums in Northern Ireland was on the authority of a Reception Order based on this section of the 1898 Act. The Statutory Regulations detailed the exact method of admission. An application for the committal of a person alleged to be of 'unsound mind' was presented by the next of kin to the local resident magistrate or justice of the peace, who then sent it (with full details of the person's residence and financial position) to the registrar in lunacy. Having received this application, the registrar sent a medical visitor to the 'person alleged to be of unsound mind', to examine him and to inform him of the application. The patient had four days within which to lodge a written objection with the registrar. The registrar then sent the initial application, the report of the medical visitor and any objections or evidence to the designated representative of the Lord Chancellor (after 1921 it became the Lord Chief Justice) who made the decision 'to make an order' or to ask for a hearing of the case. [HMSO(NI) 1930b, p. 217]; HMSO(Irl) 1904, Vol. 8, pp. 44-45)

In this way the law aimed to protect the liberty of the individual. However, the procedure was cumbersome and unpopular.

In 1921, the number of people admitted to district asylums using this procedure was 454, which formed 56 per cent of total admissions in that year. (See Table 1.3) There were a number of reasons why this figure was not higher. The serious overcrowding which had occurred in asylums throughout Ireland at the end of the nineteenth century had made asylum managers reluctant to accept new admissions. Ordinary admissions – of patients of unsound mind who were neither dangerous or criminal – could be redirected more easily to relatives or to the workhouse. (Finnane 1981, p. 101) Furthermore, relatives were reluctant to use this method of admission because of their legal obligation to pay for maintenance. According to the Lunatic Asylums (Ireland) Act 1875, Sect. 16:

> Where any person shall be confined to any district lunatic asylum as a patient, it shall be lawful for a court of summary jurisdiction, in case it shall be proved to the satisfaction of such court that such patient has an estate applicable to his maintenance and more than sufficient to maintain his family (if any), by order to require the relation or other – the person in receipt of the income of such patient, within one month after the service of such order, to pay the charges of the examination, removal, lodging, maintenance, clothing, medicine, and care of such patient, and within one month from the times in such order respectively specified, to continue to pay, so long as such patient shall remain in such district lunatic asylum, the charges which may from time to time be incurred in respect of the lodging, maintenance, clothing, medicine, and care of such patient in such district lunatic asylum.

Before 1901 the obligation on relatives to pay for the transportation of the patient to the asylum and ongoing maintenance had not applied to patients admitted as 'dangerous' or 'criminal'. In 1901 this responsibility was extended to relatives of all patients regardless of the manner of admission. [The Lunacy (Ireland) Act 1901 (1 Edw. V11, c. 17)] However, it took some time for this to affect patterns of admission.

Admission as a 'dangerous lunatic' In 1921, 343 people (42 per cent of total admissions) were admitted to asylums in Northern Ireland as dangerous lunatics. The legal basis for these admissions was the Lunacy (Ireland) Act 1867 which stipulated that persons brought before two justices 'having being discovered under circumstances denoting a derangement of mind and a purpose of committing some indictable offence' had to be examined by the district dispensary medical officer. If he certified that the person was a 'dangerous lunatic' then he/she could be taken directly to the local asylum. As we have already seen, admission to an asylum in this manner had a number of advantages for relatives. Ordinary admission procedures did not provide for the 'conveyance' of the insane person to the asylum, nor were the governors of the asylum obliged to admit the person. In addition, prior to the Lunacy (Ireland) Act 1901, relatives of a lunatic committed as a 'dangerous lunatic' could not be legally required to pay maintenance even if able to do so.

The large scale use of this admission procedure in nineteenth century Ireland has been well documented by Finnane. (1981, ch. 3) In 1890, for example, three out of every four male admissions and seven out of every ten female admissions fell into this category. Many attempts by Inspectors of Lunacy to change the situation met with failure. Not only was there little agreement among the public about what constituted dangerous lunacy, but doctors were also often unclear. (Finnane 1981, pp. 110-12) Because of the confusion between 'insanity' and 'dangerous insanity', and because of the financial advantages, this method of admission (which had the added stigma of a court appearance) continued to be a significant mode of entry to district asylums in Ireland until there was a radical change in lunacy laws in Northern Ireland in 1932 (See Figure 2.1) and in the Republic of Ireland in 1945.

Admission as a 'criminal lunatic' This admission category constituted a very small proportion of yearly admissions. These were patients who were not in need of the special security arrangements found in the Criminal Lunatic Asylum, Dublin and were financed completely from central government funds. [HMSO(NI) 1924, p. 8] Five different pieces of legislation featured in this category of admission. (See Table 1.3) The largest number of patients were admitted by Order of the Governor of Northern Ireland. Others were admitted by virtue of Army and Navy Acts which related to a person (other than a commissioned officer) about to be discharged from Her Majesty's forces and 'who was deemed to be dangerous and of unsound mind', or a person 'of unsound mind having no relative willing to take charge of him'. (Army Act 1881, Sect. 91 and Naval Settlement Act 1884, Sect. 3)

In addition, a small number of people continued to be admitted under the Poor Law Act (Scotland) 1898. This group is interesting because of what it represented. Throughout the nineteenth century there had been an ongoing battle between Poor Law officials in Ireland and those in England and Scotland because of the propensity among British officials to repatriate paupers who had any connection with Ireland, without any attempt to get the agreement of the person or to make arrangements with the Irish authorities. (Burke 1987, pp. 192-97) Irish officials were doubly dissatisfied because there were no reciprocal arrangements – English and Scottish paupers could not be repatriated from Ireland. Under Section 9 of the Poor Law Act (Scotland) 1898 a destitute person of Irish origin (who had not been resident for five years in Scotland) was automatically transferred to Ireland. While the ordinary poor person might have been simply escorted to the boat, the 'lunatic poor' were delivered to a district asylum.

Who was the law protecting ?

Early lunacy laws had been aimed at the protection of the property of the 'person of unsound mind'. Later, protection of society from potentially dangerous lunatics became an important facet of the law. Later still, protection of the interests of local councils (against unecessary expenditure) became an issue. By 1921, because of the complex nature of the laws surrounding admissions to asylums, it was extremely unclear which interests were most important. The intention of the law was that judgements by the legal authorities should be based on the patient's ability to protect himself and his property from exploitation, the possibility of his committing a criminal offence and the likelihood of his being a danger to other individuals in society.

The manner in which the law was used in admission procedures was more often based on other criteria than those intended. The financial implications of each admission had a direct bearing on the likelihood of the patient being designated as dangerous or criminal. If the relatives of a patient or the administration of the asylum could avoid the burden of contributing in whole or in part to his maintenance they had an incentive to use the law most likely to achieve this end. This led to the extraordinary situation in 1921 where more than half of the asylum population throughout Ireland had been admitted as 'dangerous lunatics'. (Finnane 1981, Ch. 3: Robins 1986, Ch. 10)

Because of the complexity of the law, it was difficult for patients and their relatives to understand the basis of confinement to an asylum. It also led to confusion in the mind of the public on the nature of mental disorder. The fact that within the asylum there was no distinction between patients who required protection from society and those who were a threat to society added to public confusion. This lack of public understanding of mental disorder increased the isolation of the asylum population from the general population and further emphasized the stigma attached to certification.

Discussion

Lunacy policies as inherited by the Northern Ireland government in 1921 reflected the history of Ireland in the 100 years prior to partition – a history of a colonized people divided by political strife and worn out by poverty and famine. Social and economic factors had determined the shape of the asylum system in terms of its size and the composition of the patient population. However, it was the particular combination of political and economic events existing at specific times which caused certain policies to emerge and others to be jettisoned. An unusual set of circumstances in early nineteenth century Ireland had led to a major policy initiative – the establishment of a network of public asylums for the 'insane poor'. A group of interested Irish MPs had capitalized on the

31

availability of public money and the highly interventionist style of the (British) government in Ireland to 'better' the lives of the poor. Later in the century, when public money again became available for the asylums, there was no political or public interest in lunacy reform. Debates which preceded the Lunacy Act 1890 in England had not extended to Ireland. As a result, the legal and administrative framework for the provision of care and treatment for the insane remained static during the later part of the nineteenth and the early part of the twentieth centuries.

In 1921 the new Ministry for Home Affairs inherited six district asylums which were overcrowded, outmoded and costly. It also inherited a set of lunacy laws which were difficult to understand and complex to administer. Just as political circumstances had dictated the initiation of a major policy change in relation to mental disorder in the early nineteenth century, so now circumstances dictated that until the question of the political position of Northern Ireland in relation to England and to the remainder of Ireland was clarified, no major changes in policy would take place. The lack of political interest in lunacy policy meant that the administration of the law and of the district asylums was left in the hands of the local government officials who had been carrying out these tasks, under the direction of the Inspectorate of Lunacy, since 1898. Pressure for change did exist. It was emerging from three sources – from local councils, from attendants' unions, and from the medical profession. However, none of these groups had any real power and the financial situation in the Province precluded the possibility of any change which involved extra expenditure. As a result, local councils found themselves administering services over which they had little control. Nursing and medical staff worked together but with vastly different ideas on what the services were meant to achieve. Patients were assured of an adequate living standard relative to the general population, but no hope of treatment. The public had shelved responsibility for the issue and politicians were deeply engaged in more serious matters of state. Unless the impetus came from outside, there was little hope of change or improvement in lunacy laws or services in Northern Ireland in the immediate future.

2 Transforming the lunacy laws – 1932

The Royal Commission on Lunacy and Mental Disorder articulated the philosophy of the major changes in mental health legislation which took place in England in 1930 (Mental Treatment Act) and in Northern Ireland [Mental Treatment Act (NI)]. 'The keynote of the past has been detention, the keynote of the future should be prevention and treatment'. (HMSO 1926, para. 42) The two Acts, though containing some similar elements, were quite different. The English Act was a short amending Act which ran alongside the Lunacy Act 1890, while the Northern Ireland Act was a major piece of legislation repealing and replacing nineteenth century laws. In England, the need for reform of the 1890 Act arose from the development of modern psychiatric practice in the early 1920s (Jones 1960, p. 103; Unsworth 1987, p. 125). As part of the United Kingdom, Northern Ireland was now exposed to the ideas and debates prevalent in England. This led to the emergence of new definitions of existing problems and to a broader view of possible solutions to these problems.

An examination of the process leading up to the passing of the Mental Treatment Act (NI) 1932 is not only interesting in terms of what it tells us about mental health policy, but also because it is a good example of the policy process at this time. During the preparation for and the implementation of the Act, one finds encapsulated many of the economic and political dilemmas of this period. These were the struggle for political and economic autonomy, the inevitable move towards policies similar to those in Britain and the effort to maintain some semblance of democratic debate in a society which was still deeply divided by religious and political affiliation. The preparatory phase for a change in the Northern Ireland law was relatively short – from 1930 to 1932 – because most of the debate had already taken place at Westminster. The implementation phase lasted until 1948, when the introduction of a comprehensive health service structure radically altered the context of mental health provision.

A new definition of the problem

Easton (1967) distinguishes between internal and external sources of policy change. In practice it is often difficult to separate these, but in the case of the Mental Treatment Act (NI) 1932 the two sets of influences were clear. Debates which originated within Northern Ireland were very different in content from those emanating in England. In Northern Ireland, local councils responsible for running the six district asylums were concerned with the financial aspects of lunacy provision. During the 1920s, the Ministry for Home Affairs was under constant pressure from Belfast Corporation to change the basis for the financing of the district asylums. As numbers of patients increased and as central funding decreased, the financial burden fell increasingly on ratepayers. The economic boom experienced immediately after the First World War quickly gave way to economic depression. In this economic climate councils had very little hope of raising extra local revenue. It was clear that without a change in central funding arrangements for district asylums improvements in services were out of the question.

However, internal pressures did not lead to change. The impetus came from England, with the passing of the 1930 Mental Treatment Act (for England and Wales). By the early twentieth century, psychiatric opinion in England favoured voluntary treatment of mental illness and emphasized the need for outpatient or non residential patient care, neither of which were provided under the 1890 Act. Public attention was focused on the lunacy question following the publication by Dr Montague Lomax of *The Experiences of an Asylum Doctor* in which he was highly critical of the care being given to patients at Prestwich Hospital, Manchester. (See Jones 1972, p. 232) In response to public anxiety about the possibility of unecessary confinement in asylums, the government in 1924 appointed a Royal Commission on Lunacy and Mental Disorder to be chaired by Hugh Pattison (later Lord) Macmillan. (Unsworth 1987, p. 186) The Macmillan Commission's recommendations emphasized the need for early treatment of mental disorder, the desirability of admission procedures which allowed treatment without certification, and the need to break the link between the Poor Law and asylum treatment by introducing a uniform procedure for paying (private) and non-paying (pauper) patients. (HMSO 1926) Members of the Commission believed that these changes would encourage people to seek early treatment without fear of long term confinement to an institution.

Most of the recommendations of the Commission were relevent to Northern Ireland with one major exception which is worth highlighting. Asylums throughout Ireland had always had a separate administrative structure from that of the Poor Law and patients did not have to be classified as paupers to be admitted to a publicly funded district asylum. Except for those transferred from workhouses, most patients were admitted on the application of a relative rather than that of a Relieving Officer. This aspect of the Irish system had been commended by the Minority Report of the Royal Commission on the Poor Law 1909. [HMSO 1909, Vol.3, p. 243] It meant that public provision for the mentally ill in Northern Ireland during the 1920s was not subject to the main criticism levelled at similar provisions in England – that of unecessarily adding the stigma of pauperism to that of insanity. However, though workhouses and asylums were administratively separate, poverty and admission to an asylum were often linked together. The asylum population throughout Ireland had been dominated by the 'labouring classes' during the nineteenth century (Finnane 1981, p. 134), a trend that continued into the early twentieth century. [PRO(NI) HOS 14/1/2/1-5; HOS 28/1/1/13-16]

The focus on mental disorder as illness formed a central theme in the Report of the Macmillan Commission. Developments in medical practice resulted in growing optimism regarding the possibility of curing conditions which previously had been perceived as incurable. It followed from this that early and easy access to treatment would enhance the chance of recovery and therefore the law should ideally facilitate rather than hinder this access. In Northern Ireland, none of these debates were evident in any of the reports of the period, though the Inspectors of Lunacy, Dr W. R. Dawson and Dr N. C. Patrick, were undoubtedly aware of developments taking place in England. Their reports, however, continued to be written in the language and style of their predecessors. Similarly, these new ideas were not evident in the major local government report of the period – that of the Departmental Commission on Local Government Administration in Northern Ireland (1924-26). [HMSO(NI) 1927]

This commission, chaired by Professor R. J. Johnstone MP, an eminent Belfast surgeon, was appointed to examine the 'suitability, efficiency and cost' of the current administrative structures of local government, public health, the Poor Law, and the district asylums. It was asked to make recommendations which would increase efficiency without 'creating unecessary additional burdens on the local rates or on public funds'. [HMSO(NI) 1927, p. 2] The Commission praised the district asylums for their economic efficiency. (Ibid. paras. 248-250] It was clear in their report that the asylum system compared favourably with workhouses, which were seen as uneconomic and unsuitable for the range of patients being housed there in the 1920s. The Commission did recognize the 'specialized nature' of the work being done within the asylums and recommended the appointment of a special expert committee on lunacy law. (Ibid. para. 299)

A three man committee was appointed in 1929 to advise the Minister of Home Affairs on necessary changes in the lunacy laws. The members – the Chief Medical Officer, Lt Col. W. R. Dawson, and the Resident Medical Superintendents of Belfast and Down Asylums, Dr S. J. Graham and Dr N. J. Nolan – were supported in their efforts to bring about reform by the psychiatrists working in the six district asylums. [PRO(NI) CAB 9B/176/1] As members of the Royal Medico Psychological Association (RMPA) these doctors were part of a wider professional network and must have been aware of the inadequacy of the system in Northern Ireland. Annual meetings of the RMPA during this period showed the diversity of opinion within the medical profession on what constituted mental disorder. This was the heyday of discussion on possible treatments – ranging from surgery to psychotherapy. There were as many different perceptions on mental disorders as there were speakers at conferences.

Dr Richard Leaper, Medical Superintendent at St. Patricks Hospital, Dublin, speaking at the Annual General Meeting of the RMPA in 1931 was very clear about his own viewpoint.

> Nine out of ten forms of mental disease are due to the ever varying vagaries of hereditary defect . . . I believe insane inheritance, or the outcome of the unions of neurotics, the feeble minded and psychopaths, to be the real and everlasting reason for the numbers of the insane population in the world today. (Leaper 1931, p. 683)

Leaper felt that though advances had been made in treatment, psychiatry had failed to make any real impact on recovery rates – and therefore had achieved nothing. Other psychiatrists were more optimistic. Dr A. R. Martin, an Ulsterman working in the USA, expressed hope about the move towards a more holistic view of man. In a review of recent developments in psychiatry, he saw 'a shift from static to dynamic concepts, from dualism to monism, from mechanism to vitalism, from what is objective to what is subjective.' (Martin 1935, p. 148) He regarded treatments on the basis of physical causes alone as a waste of time but was optimistic about the psychotherapeutic approaches. More important than the actual approaches, was what he saw as a positive approach to the treatment of mental disorder.

> The new dynamic philosophies and psycho-biological concepts have at least shown us the way to break down that unwholesome, despairing and fatalistic attitude that too long has persisted towards mental illness. (Martin 1935, p. 153)

Martin was not working in Northern Ireland, but his article was published in the Ulster Medical Journal – a journal which very rarely had a contribution from a psychiatrist. Psychiatry was still very much on the periphery of medicine in Northern Ireland, and the handful of doctors working in asylums continued to be isolated from their colleagues in general medicine. Debates on changing concepts of mental disorder were only central to the few doctors directly engaged in practice. These doctors, working in poor conditions and overwhelmed by increasing patient numbers, had little influence on the direction of mental health policies either at local or central level. The impetus for the acceptance of an official definition of lunacy based on a medical rather than a legal model came from England. This redefinition meant that existing solutions to the problems of lunacy – both legal and administrative – were no longer acceptable. A reformulation of the problems caused by mental disorder within a health care model called for new solutions based on that model.

Shaping policy

Although the Departmental Commission on Local Government Administration in Northern Ireland (1924-27) had recommended that a special committee to advise on lunacy reform be set up immediately, it was not until July 1930 that Parliamentary discussion on the subject began. During that same month the Mental Treatment Act (for England and Wales) had received the Royal Assent. Between then and June 1932 (when the Mental Treatment Act (NI) became law) discussions took place within the Ministry for Home Affairs, during Parliamentary Debates and at local council level. There is little evidence of consultation between the Ministry and professional bodies or other organizations – probably because of the relatively underdeveloped state of psychiatry and mental nursing in Northern Ireland at the time, and the lack of general interest in what was seen as a local government problem.

When the time came for the preparation of a new law, the enormity of the task became clear. Not only had Britain passed a Lunacy Act in 1890, but it also had Mental Deficiency Acts in 1913 and 1927 and another Mental Treatment Act in 1930. Although Northern Ireland could and did benefit from the discussions which had taken place in preparation for each new piece of British legislation, it had nevertheless to replace a set of legal procedures based on nineteenth century assumptions about mental disorder by one based on the changing assumptions of the 1930s.

Certain themes emerged at different stages of the debates – some of which were incorporated in the final draft of the Bill. These were the need for separate institutions for people suffering from a mental defect; the need for a uniform method of admission to district asylums; the importance of providing early treatment for all forms of mental disorder; the need to break the link between treatment and certification, and between treatment and the Poor Law; and lastly the need for a new system of funding for district asylums. The need for separate specialized accommodation for people with a mental defect, was ignored by the Ministry for Home Affairs during this period, in spite of pressure from politicians and local councils. [PRO(NI) CAB 9B/176/1, letter 23 April 1931; NIHC Deb. 1932, Cols. 572 & 585] Management committees and Medical Superintendents of district asylums were united in the view that children particularly, should not be admitted to asylums. [PRO(NI) HOS 28/1/1/16] However, because there was no money available for initiatives of any kind, nothing was done to change the situation. The other themes can be subsumed under two main headings: 1) the legal implications of the changing perception of insanity as illness; and 2) the inadequacy of funding arrangements for asylums.

Insanity as illness – legal implications

The Annual Report of the Board of Control (for England and Wales) for 1918 was the first to articulate the perspective which became the major influence on the direction of law and services for mental disorder in the United Kingdom thoughout this century. This perspective placed mental disorder squarely within an 'illness' framework. Physical and mental illnesses were of a similar nature, with the possibility of treatment and cure. (HMSO 1918) This theme was later expanded by the Macmillan Commission (1924-26) which argued for a radical change in attitude towards mental disorder.

> There is no clear line of demarcation between mental and physical illness ... a mental illness may have physical concomitants and probably it always has, though they may be difficult of detection. A physical illness, on the other hand, may have and probably always has, mental concomitants. And there are many cases in which it is a question whether the physical or mental symptoms predominate. (HMSO 1926, para. 38)

The philosophy underlying this statement was that of the emerging psychiatric profession. The work of the Maudsley Hospital (opened in 1915 for shellshock cases and in 1923 for all) and that of the Tavistock Clinic (opened in 1920) were quick to gain international recognition. At the same time post-graduate training in psychological medicine became a requisite for senior medical staff in mental hospitals in Great Britain, with courses at five universities. (Jones 1960, p. 98)

Not since the heyday of moral management in the early nineteenth century had there been such optimism about the possibility of restoring people with mental disorders to full health. The Lunacy Act 1890 may have contained safeguards against the possibility of unecessary detention, but in so doing, it militated against easy access to new treatments. The new Mental Treatment Act 1930 was built on a belief in the effectiveness of psychiatric treatment. This was reflected in the language used, in the introduction of voluntary and temporary methods of admission to mental hospital (Sections 1-5) and in the inclusion of statutory powers given to local authorities to establish outpatient clinics. [Section 6(3)]

In Northern Ireland there were no parallel developments in psychiatric training or practice. District asylums continued to 'contain' rather than treat over 4,000 patients. By 1932 there was only one outpatient clinic, run by Dr N. Graham of the Belfast Asylum, at the Royal Victoria Hospital. [PRO(NI) HOS 28/1/1/15] Because many of the senior medical staff of the district asylums were members of the Royal Medico Psychological Association (RMPA) they were indeed aware of developments in England. Therefore when the opportunity arose to develop services within a medical framework, the profession used it to full advantage to enhance its professional position. The three doctors who formed the special Advisory Committee (on lunacy reform) to the Minister for Home Affairs, clearly agreed with the direction of policy change contained in the British law. For the first cabinet discussion on proposed changes in the law, the Advisory Committee had prepared a paper recommending that the general principles of the English Mental Treatment Act be adopted for Northern Ireland. [PRO(NI) CAB 9B/176/1] This meeting took place on 7 July 1930, just three days before the English Act received Royal Assent. The Cabinet accepted the recommendations of the Advisory Committee and approved the drafting of the new legislation in accordance with these recommendations. These included proposals for changes in designation of staff and of institutions – from 'asylum' to 'mental hospital', from 'attendant' to 'nurse'; the introduction of voluntary and temporary periods of treatment; and the extension of the control of the Ministry for Home Affairs over local asylum committees of management in relation to numbers, qualification and salaries of staff. [PRO(NI) CAB 9B/176/1]

When the Mental Treatment Bill came before the Northern Ireland Parliament for the Second Reading on 23 March 1932, there was general acceptance of the 'treatment model' as contained in the draft legislation. Sir R. Dawson Bates, Minister for Home Affairs, established the framework for discussion in his introductory remarks. 'Mental disease, like other forms of disease, is in many cases curable and the chances of effecting a cure are infinitely improved if treatment is undertaken in the incipient stages of the disease'. [NIHC Deb. 1932, Col. 548] The proposal to abolish terms such as 'lunatic' and 'asylum', was welcomed by Richard Byrne (MP for Falls, Belfast), who thought lunatic asylum a 'horrible name for an institution'. (Ibid. Col. 570) The majority of participants in the debate spoke in terms of prevention, treatment and cure of mental patients and accepted the removal of mental disorder from a framework dominated by legal protectionism to one guided by medical opinion. However, some of the MPs showed that their understanding of mental disorder was sometimes limited. John Beattie (Labour MP for Pottinger, Belfast) regaled the House with stories aimed at convincing his listeners that no mentally ill person would look for treatment voluntarily as this would be an admission of 'derangement'.

> A mentally deranged man always thinks the man beside him is the one who is mentally deranged. I heard a story about a prominent leader of the Unionist Party visiting Purdysburn. He was going through a ward with a doctor and the doctor said to him: "That gentleman is going out tomorrow". He went over to the man and said: "Good-day my friend". The patient said: "Good-day and who might you be?". "I am the Lord Hugh Cecil", he replied. The patient said: " You will not be long here till they cure you that disease. When I came here I thought I was the Duke of York". (NIHC Deb. 1932, Col. 562)

Beattie warned the Minister that he was making a mistake in setting up outpatient clinics. 'The other point to which I want to draw the attention of the Minister is that if he thinks any person is going to go for extern treatment for mental disease, he is greatly mistaken'. (Ibid.) Beattie may not have understood all of the concepts but at least he was in favour of the Bill in general. Others objected to it because of what it represented politically. Cahir Healy (Nationalist MP for South Fermanagh) thought the Bill

> . . . one of those Measures to which no objection could be taken, I think, on any side of the house, but equally it is not of an urgent character . . . I think the reason for the introduction of this Measure is not that anybody here wants it – the Government do not want it – but that a similar Measure was introduced in the Imperial parliament, and this craze you have got of walking step by step with Britain impelled you to introduce legislation on almost identical lines. (NIHC Deb. 1932, Col. 573)

The Bill was passed to the Senate for discussion in May 1932. Here the new definition of mental disorder was made explicit.

> One of the chief objects of this Bill is to emphasize the fact that persons suffering from mental disease and cared for in mental

40

hospitals are invalids suffering from afflictions of the mind, and are just as blameless and deserving of every sympathy as persons in hospitals suffering from or treated for afflictions of the body ... Unfortunately, the procedure followed in sending persons of unsound mind to asylums in Ireland has rather tended to give ordinary persons the impression that they are committed as criminals, but as a result of this Bill it is hoped that the idea that to be of unsound mind is a criminal offence will die out. (NI Senate Deb. 1932, Cols. 177-178]

By implication it was assumed that the extension of medical powers and the contraction of judicial procedures would result in a less stigmatizing service which would, in turn, remove the stigma from the condition itself.

When it became law on 7 June 1932 the Mental Treatment Act (NI) contained the basis for the new approach to mental disorder. It introduced the possibility of a voluntary admission for treatment.

Any person who is desirous of voluntarily submitting himself to treatment for illness of a mental or kindred nature and who makes a written application for that purpose ... may be received and maintained as a voluntary patient. (Section 1)

This patient could leave the hospital after giving seventy-two hours notice in writing. The possibility of receiving treatment for a mental illness on a voluntary basis was not an entirely new idea. Throughout the nineteenth century it had been the practice for patients in private asylums to be admitted as voluntary boarders but this had not been allowed in the public system because of the fear of unecessary public expenditure. Now it was accepted that early treatment of a minor disorder might lead to an improvement or cure of the condition and thus to early discharge.

While the procedure to allow admission to hospital treatment on a voluntary basis was aimed at encouraging medical intervention at an early stage in the development of a mental illness, the procedure allowing for 'temporary' admission was aimed at patients suffering from serious disorders due to curable physical causes. These were patients who were not able to appreciate the need for treatment and were not likely to go into hospital voluntarily. The Northern Ireland Act differed from the English Act in one important respect. This was the use of the criterion 'likely to benefit by treatment' for patients being admitted on a temporary basis. As Dr T. W. H. Weir (Medical Inspector, Mental Health) pointed out to his colleagues at a meeting of the Royal Medico Psychological Association held in Dublin, 'this opened the portal of entry under this temporary category much wider'. (Weir 1949, p. 696) The application for temporary admission could be made by a relative or a Relieving Officer and had to be accompanied by two medical certificates. (Section 4) A temporary admission was for an initial period of six months but could be extended for further three monthly periods. [Section 4 (11) and (12)] As in the case of voluntary admissions, this was a major step forward.

There is another interesting difference in this section of the law as it was introduced in England and Northern Ireland. In England the strong link between the Poor Law structures and the public asylum system had meant that, prior to 1930, all admissions to asylums were made by the Relieving Officer of the local Poor Law Union. In order to streamline the procedures for all patients (then designated 'rate-aided' and 'private') an application for temporary treatment could (after 1930) be made by either a relative or a Relieving Officer, without reference to the financial status of the patient. In the English Mental Treatment Act 1930, the Relieving Officer received the title of the 'duly authorized officer of the local authority'. [Section 5(2)] In Northern Ireland, where most applications for admissions to asylums were made by patients' relatives, it did not seem necessary to make this distinction explicit, so the Relieving Officer retained the nineteenth century title. Interestingly, the trend in applications for hospital admission continued to follow the pattern already established in each country. In Northern Ireland relatives have been more likely (than Relieving/Welfare Officers) to apply for admission of a patient to mental hospital while the situation in England has been the reverse. (Herron 1990; Hoyle and Hawksworth 1956; Sheppard 1990, p. 3)

The possibility of being certified as a 'person of unsound mind' remained in the new legislation. The new procedure was called a 'reception order' to be signed by a Resident Magistrate or a Justice of the Peace and accompanied by one medical certificate. [Mental Treatment Act (NI) 1932, Section 9] Again the application could be made either by a relative or by a Relieving Officer. (Section 10) A number of safeguards were built into the procedure to ensure that no patient would be unecesssarily confined under this section of the Act. This included a designated time period for the order (one year followed by 2-3 years) and an obligation on the Resident Medical Superintendent to inform the patient of his or her right to be visited by an independent Resident Magistrate.(Sections 13 and 18) The English Act did not include details of reception orders as these were already in force under the Lunacy Act 1890. (Sections 4-8)

The introduction of this single reception order for patients judged as in need of long-term care within the newly designated mental hospitals, brought to an end different admission procedures in use prior to 1932. (See Tables 1.2 and 1.3) The classification of 'dangerous lunatic' finally disappeared. The continued use of judicial procedures for reception orders was seen as necessary in order to safeguard the 'liberty of the subject'.

> Taking the Bill as a whole, I think that the House will agree that the liberty of the subject has been carefully protected throughout, and that is one of the most important matters in dealing with cases of mental patients. (NIHC Deb. 1932, Col. 185)

Although incorporating these safeguards for long-term patients the Act focused, not on the judicial aspects of confinement, but rather on the importance of regarding mental disorder as an illness capable of treatment and cure.

Local or central funding?

The second major theme which emerged during the preparation for the passing of the Mental Treatment Act (NI) 1932, was the need for increased funding to the local councils responsible for administering the asylums. The decision in 1923 to pay a fixed grant of £37,079 per year (the average of the preceding three years capitation grant) was highly unpopular with local councils experiencing severe financial difficulties. Between 1923 and 1930 the shortfall between central funding and asylum costs, a shortfall which had to be funded from local rates, continued to increase.

Because of pressure from local councils Sir R. Dawson Bates, Minister for Home Affairs, frequently brought the issue before the Northern Ireland Cabinet. [PRO(NI) CAB 9B/176/1] On the 7 July 1930, in a Cabinet paper outlining the proposed changes in lunacy laws, he argued that the existing grant to asylums was inequitable and inelastic. Over a year later, in October 1931, when preparation for the new Mental Treatment Bill (NI) was underway, the Minister proposed that the Cabinet approve a return to the principle of capitation payments. A proposed per capita payment of five shillings per week would cost £58,500 on the basis of 4,500 patients – the average number under treatment in the Province. He urged the Cabinet to reject the proposals made by the Leslie Committee (set up to examine financial relations between central and local government) which acknowledged the problem of underfunding to district asylums and proposed the proposed abolition of central funds for dispensaries and workhouses and redeployment of these funds to asylums. [HMSO(NI) 1931, pp. 67 & 115] In spite of his efforts to have a decision on the matter included in the new mental health law, Dawson Bates failed to convince the Cabinet that any change should be made in the method of financing district asylums until the issue of the relationship between central and local government funding of public services was satisfactorily resolved.

This decision has to be seen within the context of a world-wide depression which was having a severe effect on the Northern Ireland economy. In 1930 and 1931 the Province experienced the sharp edge of the depression due to a fall in the value of products, a fall in exports, and a rise in unemployment. (Kennedy and Ollerenshaw 1985, p. 191) The Ministry of Finance was determined to curtail expenditure in all areas by limiting any expansion or changes in services which might require additional government funding. [PRO(NI) CAB 9A/3/1] As an alternative solution to the problem, some members of the Northern Ireland Parliament were in favour of exploring the possibility of an annual contribution from the United Kingdom Parliament. This was opposed by the Minister of Finance, Hugh Pollock, who stood firm in his position. There was uproar as the Bill was debated in both Houses of the Northern Ireland Parliament. The way in which it was worded (Clause 54) made the financial position of the asylums even more precarious than it had been before.

> The Ministry shall, by regulations made with approval of the Ministry of Finance, provide for the payment out of moneys provided by Parliament, to each council of a county or county borough, in respect of the expenses of the council on account of the maintenance of rate-aided patients in the public mental hospital established for such county or county borough, of annual grants of such amounts and subject to such conditions as may be prescribed in the regulations, and such regulations may provide for the discontinuance of grants payable to such a county or county borough council under Section 10 of the Local Government Act (NI) 1923 . . . (NIHC Deb. 1932, Col. 580)

As many MPs pointed out, this left the financing of asylums at the mercy of the Minister of Finance. As a result of the opposition to its inclusion, this clause was omitted when the Bill came before the Senate for its Second Reading in May 1932. The Act, when passed, did not make any reference to financial arrangements for the administration of the asylums. Neither did it contain any clauses which might involve new money. Particularly significant was the absence of any local authority power to develop locally based services. The English legislation gave local authorities powers to provide outpatient clinics and aftercare services; to encourage voluntary organisations concerned with the prevention and treatment of mental illness; and to fund research into mental illness. [Mental Treatment Act 1930, Sect 6(3)] No such element was included in the Northern Ireland Act

The decision to avoid any additional public expenditure and the discussions leading up to it can be seen as reflecting the two different approaches to government which existed within the Northern Ireland Parliament at this time. (See Bew, Gibbon and Patterson 1979, p. 76) The 'populist' approach, represented by Dawson Bates, favoured parity with Great Britain in public and social services, while the 'anti-populists', represented by Pollock, favoured stringency. [PRO(NI) D 1022/2/22] Pollock won and the outcome was a new piece of legislation which did not even attempt to address the issue which was of prime importance to those involved in services for mentally ill people in Northern Ireland.

The implementation of the new law

The most important elements in the new Act were : 1) The replacement of the language of lunacy and vagrancy by the language of mental illness and disorder, the former derived from concepts of social control and the latter from concepts of care and treatment. 2) The introduction of new procedures for admission to treatment. (Parts 1 & 2) The most important of these was the procedure for Voluntary admission, which emphasized the similarily betweeen mental and physical illness. The other new procedure, for a Temporary admission, counteracted the notion of permanency implied by certification. Certification of a person (as being of unsound mind) would only be necessary for a small proportion of patients rather than for everyone undergoing treatment for a mental disorder, as had been the case prior to 1932. 3) The extension of treatment for mental disorder outside of the mental hospital. (Part 4) Though worded in such a way as to prevent an interpretation which might lead to new expenditure, the Act introduced the concept of treatment after discharge (extern treatment) either in a clinic or in the home of the patient, and also for the first time allowed for the boarding out of patients in a private hospital or 'approved house'.

Admission patterns

The immediate impact of the new Act was on admission procedures to the six district asylums now redesignated as mental hospitals. Voluntary, temporary and certified admissions replaced the earlier categories of admission – as a 'person of unsound mind', as a 'dangerous lunatic' or as a 'criminal lunatic'. During the period before this change took place, the pattern of admissions had already begun to alter as is shown in the following diagram. There was an overall increase in admissions, explained by an increase in patients of 'unsound mind', a decrease in admissions of 'dangerous' lunatics and a relatively stable (if small) number of admissions as 'criminal' lunatics.

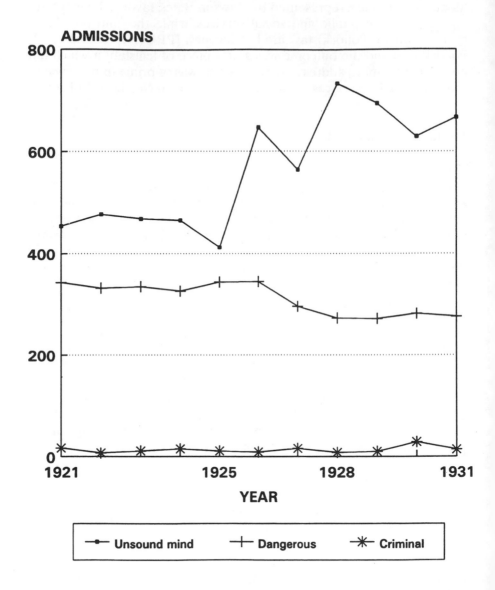

Figure 2.1   Legal status of admissions to district asylums 1921-31

Source: Government Statistics

During the years immediately following the introduction of the Mental Treatment Act (NI) 1932, the total number of patients being admitted to mental hospitals did not change very much. But within this the pattern of admission changed radically, with voluntary and temporary admission procedures being used immediately by a significant number of patients and a steady decline in certified admissions. During the war years and these trends continued though there was a dramatic decline in overall admissions. The relationship between war and mental health statistics has been the subject of academic debate for many years. (Lewis 1941; Hemphill 1941; Dohan 1966; Fraser 1971) The drop in admissions to mental hospitals during war years has been associated with the absorbtion of aggression, or with the strengthening of group identity in the face of a common enemy. Since Northern Ireland was peripheral to the war effort and since there was only one serious bombing incident during this time, this is not a plausible explanation for the drop in admissions. Perhaps it had more to do with practical considerations. As Belfast Mental Hospital was designated as an Emergency Hospital, 500 of its patients transferred to the other hospitals in 1941. [HMSO(NI) 1948a, p. 48] It is most likely that those hospitals (which already considered themselves overcrowded) controlled their admissions fairly strictly during this period. Figure 2.2 shows the emerging patterns of admissions.

Convinced that this was the way forward, the Ministry for Home Affairs encouraged the use of both voluntary and temporary admission procedures but there were immediate problems with both. [HMSO(NI) 1948a, pp. 49-50] In relation to voluntary admissions the question arose as to how long a patient should be allowed to remain as a voluntary patient if his or her mental state deteriorated. Some hospitals were in favour of allowing any patient admitted in a voluntary capacity to remain so regardless of his or her subsequent mental state. The Ministry, however, disagreed with this view.

> . . . the Act can be interpreted only as specifying that a patient can be maintained on a voluntary basis only so long as he is able to express a wish to remain in that class and appreciates his rights as a voluntary patient. Should be permanently depart from these standards then he should no longer be maintained as a voluntary patient. [HMSO(NI) 1948a, p. 49]

The problems with temporary admission procedures were more difficult to overcome. Surprisingly these problems were described in some detail in the report of the Ministry. (Ibid. p. 51) In all likelihood this was an effort by Dr T. W. H. Weir (Medical Inspector, Mental Health) to educate his colleagues.

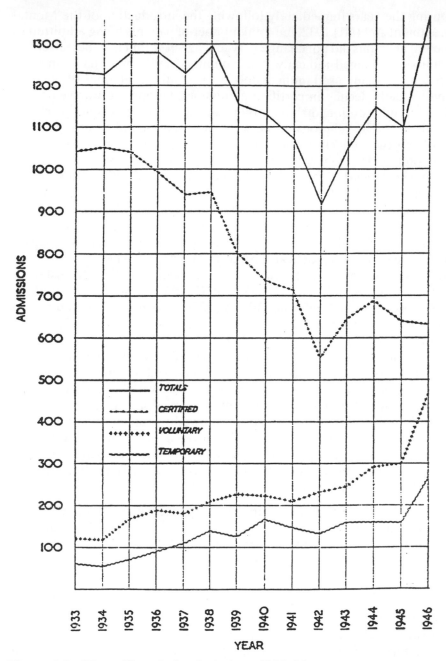

Figure 2.2   Mental hospitals admissions 1933-46

Source: HMSO (NI) 1948a, p. 54

The main problem stemmed from the lack of competence among GPs in making a decision about the type of mental disorder and the probable pattern of recovery for any given patient. According to the Ministry, there were clear criteria for admission as a temporary patient.

> The temporary category is essentially to provide for mentally ill persons who, with treatment, are likely to recover within the course of six months, or in some cases a year. It was never intended as a means of sparing patients or relatives the need for certification where such was necessary. Therefore, persons suffering from senile dementia, gross organic brain changes, or any other mental disorder of an irrecoverable nature should not come within the scope of the temporary grade as it exists at present. [HMSO(NI) 1948a, p. 51]

Not only were some patients suitable for certification being admitted as temporary patients, but the opposite was also happening. According to the Ministry, many certified patients admitted between 1933 and 1946 were discharged 'as recovered' within a year of admission and 'these patients should have been given the benefit of temporary status and thereby have avoided legal certification. (Ibid) Full advantage was not being taken of the temporary admission procedure and more patients than necessary were involved in judicial proceedings. One reason for this was obviously the lack of knowledge of mental disorder on the part of GPs. However, there was another more practical reason which was probably more important. An application for temporary admission required two medical certificates while certification involved a 'reception order' signed by a Resident Magistrate plus one medical certificate. In rural areas, because it was particularly difficult to find two doctors, it was often more convenient to use the judicial procedure regardless of the stigma involved.

Treatment

Changes in admission classification did not necessarily imply any changes in care or treatment within the hospitals, although there was a growing awareness among psychiatrists of the need to develop modern psychiatric treatments. The Down Mental Hospital was regarded as progressive in its approach and its records offer some good examples of what was happening during the 1920s and 1930s. In 1925 Dr M. J. Nolan, Resident Medical Superintendent, wrote under the heading of 'medical and moral treatment': 'The keynote is hospitalization, segregation of the mental classes, and suitable recreation and occupation to the widest possible extent'. (Down 1925, p. xiii) In the following year, he wrote that he was encouraged by the fact that the three main elements of moral treatment 'discipline, order and employment' were now in evidence in all of the wards of his hospital.

> It is indeed of striking interest to note that so many individuals whose actions unfitted them for ordinary social life, have yet sufficient of the herd instinct left intact to enable them to live in harmonious association, and to exhibit an extraordinary tolerance to each others peculiarities. (Down 1926, p. xv)

By 1930 plans for new medical and moral treatments were in place. Medical advances would include equipment for 'electro-medical and hydro-therapeutic treatment' and moral treatment would include an occupational therapy room – a room set aside for 'non-essential work'. (Down 1930, p. xvi) These plans reflected two strands of medical thinking on mental disorder of the time. One of these emphasized the value of social treatments and the other that of physical treatments. Social treatments were based on some of the concepts of moral management from the nineteenth century and influenced by the psycho analytic school and by the work of people like Dr Adolf Meyer. (Gelder 1991: Pines 1991) Developments in physical treatments were based on the assumption that all mental disorders were due to some physical cause. Physical treatments in the form of baths, laxatives and swinging chairs had been in use since the earliest days of the treatment of madness and the end of the nineteenth century saw the emerging ideas on which both psychosurgery and shock therapies were based. However, it was not until the early part of the twentieth century that the technology became available to develop these and other treatments. (Berrios 1991: Clare 1987, ch. 6 & 7)

Dr Nolan, like many of his colleagues, was convinced of the value of occupational therapy in spite of the fact that they found it impossible to employ qualified staff until the mid 1940s. He wrote of its benefits in the casenotes of a woman patient, Cynthia Smyth.

> Instead of worrying everyone around her as to the murder of her relations, the despoliation of all her goods and chattels, and the miseries she has been subjected to by confiscation, she is now constantly getting fresh designs for all varied classes of fancy work and executes them in an excellent manner.(Down 1930, p. xvi)

During the early 1930s, new buildings for electro and hydro therapy and occupational therapy were opened at the Down Mental Hospital and in the late 1930s treatment was further extended to include the use of Cardiazol and malarial treatment. (Parkinson 1969, p. 9)

Malarial treatment was one of the physical treatments which gained and lost popularity in a very short space of time. It had been used for General Paralysis of the Insane (GPI) at Belfast Mental Hospital since

1924 when Professor York MD from the Liverpool Institute of Tropical Medicine was invited to demonstrate this treatment. [PRO(NI) HOS 28/1/1/14] The hospital became the regional centre for malarial treatment although very soon other hospitals showed an interest in carrying it out themselves. [PRO(NI) HOS 14/1/1/5] Malarial treatment became outmoded with the intoduction of antibiotics and the decrease in the number of GPI cases.

The other new treatments gaining popularity in Europe at the time – insulin therapy and electric therapy (ECT) – were not introduced in Northern Ireland until the mid 1940s. Though many doctors saw them as representing a major breakthrough in the treatment of mental disorder, some like Dr D. B. M. Lothian (RMS Down) were more sceptical. He argued that treatment would only work if 'directed to the total situation'. None of the techniques on offer could provide the complete answer – not the 'elimination of toxic foci, prolonged narcosis, insulin, cardiazol, electric shock therapy or pre-frontal leucotomy'. (Down 1942, p. ix) Lothian called for a preventive approach to mental welfare, for child guidance clinics, mental outpatient departments and provision for the treatment of the neuroses. (Ibid)

None of these services existed in Northern Ireland at the time. The Ministry was particularly anxious to develop outpatient clinics, but before 1944 there was only one outpatient clinic in operation – that at the Royal Victoria Hospital, run from the Belfast Mental Hospital. In 1944 four more clinics were opened, and by 1947 all six mental hospitals had outpatient clinics. [HMSO(NI) 1948a, p. 62] In effect, until the late 1940s, the care and treatment received by the majority of patients in mental hospitals in Northern Ireland was very similar to that of the late nineteenth century. Apart from the changes in procedures for admission to hospital, the Mental Treatment Act (NI) 1932 made no impact on this care or treatment. This was due not only to the lack of qualified staff but to the severe financial problems being experienced within the mental hospital system.

Money matters

By 1932, local councils (established in 1898) had grown accustomed to being in almost total control of health services such as the district asylums. The Lunacy Inspectorate, based within the Ministry for Home Affairs, had a monitoring function but very little power to effect any change in the standards of care or treatment. The main reason for the lack of central control was related to the system of financing of the asylums. Central funding amounted to only 16 per cent of the total income of the six district asylums in 1932. [HMSO(NI) 1933, p. 47] With this low level of central funding, policy decisions could not be imposed on local councils.

When the Mental Treatment Act (NI) 1932 was passed, councils were deeply disappointed by the fact that their financial crisis had been ignored. The Minister's prediction of a new era in treatment for mentally ill people was seen as empty rhetoric . In 1936 the Belfast Corporation intensified its campaign to alter the situation, by sending its entire Finance Committee as a delegation to the Minister for Home Affairs. [PRO(NI) CAB 9B/176/1]

Convinced by their argument the Minister, Dawson Bates, wrote to Hugh Pollock, Minister of Finance on the 16th September 1936 (five days after the Corporation delegation). In his letter he went over old ground, proposing a return to the principle of capitation grants based on fifty percent of patient costs. Basing his projected costing on actual expenditure per patient for the (which ranged from £30 in Armagh district Asylum to £44 in Omagh), he estimated the total cost as being £86,706.10s.0d. This was an increase of 134 per cent on existing funding. (Ibid) For individual hospitals it would mean increases ranging from 87 per cent at Armagh Mental Hospital to 186 per cent at Belfast Mental Hospital.

In November 1936 he sent a paper on the same subject to the Cabinet Secretariat for immediate discussion. In it he presented a strong case for the acceptance of his proposals. He also stated that he could not agree to the abolition of other local authority grants to workhouses and dispensaries as proposed by the Leslie Committee in 1931. [HMSO(NI) 1931, pp. 115-16] The proposal was never presented to the Cabinet for discussion. In September 1936, after receiving the initial proposal, Sir Wilfred B. Spender, Secretary to the Minister of Finance, wrote a lengthy argument to Sir Charles Blackmore, Cabinet Secretary, on the delicacy of the issue of payment of an additional £50,000. The nature of the financial relationship between Northern Ireland and Great Britain was such that additional central funding to local authorities was not feasable. He also reminded Blackmore that the policy of the Ministry of Finance was to follow the principle being applied in England and Wales – that of placing responsibility on local authorities for social and health services. [PRO(NI) CAB 9B/176/1]

Blackmore, convinced by Spender's argument, did not bring the issue to a full Cabinet meeting. In an effort to resolve the issue, the Prime Minister, Sir J. Craig, called a special meeting of the Ministries involved. It was attended by Dawson Bates (Home Affairs), Blackmore (Cabinet Secretary) and two senior civil servants from Finance, Duggan and Magill as well as Craig himself. Hugh Pollock, Minister of Finance, was conspicuous by his absence from this meeting, but his representatives were well prepared for the battle which ensued. As the basis for discussion Duggan presented a detailed proposal which would increase the grant to mental hospitals without incurring extra central government expenditure. The proposal could be summarized as follows : The Ministry for Home Affairs would agree to the following : 1) Increase the grant to mental hospitals to 40 per cent of net expenditure with a maximum limit in certain cases; 2) Relieve local authorities in rural and urban areas of any liability for levy for unemployment assistance due to start in April 1938, and to materially reduce the levy in Belfast and possibly Derry. (Estimated amount £34,000); 3) Relieve local authorities of liability for future quinquennial revaluation. (Estimated at £6,000 per annum); 4) Offset the cost of this, by abolishing the existing workhouses officers salaries grant, the Union medical expenditure grant, and three other small grants for local services which would amount in total to £59,709. [PRO(NI) CAB 9B/176/1, Meeting 13 Jan. 1937]

Discussion centred on the urgency of the need for additional funding for asylums in the light of the government decision not to give any extra money to local authorities. Because it was evident to Dawson Bates (Home Affairs) that no extra cash was forthcoming, he agreed that the proposal from the Ministry of Finance, as outlined by Duggan, be put to local authorities. He made it clear, however, that he objected in principle to the removal of grants to the public health services (workhouses etc). Dawson Bates was right in thinking that a re-allocation of money between local authority services was not what councils had in mind. They rejected the proposal from the Ministry of Finance and continued to campaign for extra funding.

In April 1937, just three months after the meeting involving the Prime Minister, Pollock (Finance) wrote again to Dawson Bates expressing his regret at the 'unreasonable' attitude of the councils and the 'unhelpful tactics' of the Belfast Corporation. He said he could not agree to a substantial increase in central funding to mental hospitals. He argued that block grants in Britain were no higher than in Northern Ireland and that local authorities in the remainder of the United Kingdom were bearing the burden of greater expenditure than their counterparts in Northern Ireland. Two days later Dawson Bates wrote his final letter on the matter accepting the situation with disappointment. A situation of stalemate had been reached and local councils were powerless to change it. Three years later the block grant was increased to £60,000 [Local Government (Finance) Act (NI) 1940] but this did not solve the problem and the debate continued until there was a further increase in the block grant to £90,000 in 1945. [Local Government (Finance) Act (NI) 1945] The situation was not finally resolved until the mental hospitals were integrated into the new comprehensive health services structure in 1948 when control of all hospitals passed completely out of the hands of local authorities.

This detailed acount of the wranglings over finance have been included here to illustrate the nature of the relationship between the Ministry of Home Affairs and local councils during the 1930s. Within this context it was impossible for the Ministry to make any demands on councils to improve mental health services either in terms of raising standards of treatment and care by the employment of professionally qualified staff, or by the initiation of new services such as outpatient clinics and after care facilities. The only policy implementation which could be required was a change in admission procedures, which was purely administrative. The letter of the law was indeed implemented but not the spirit of the Macmillan Commission as implied by that law.

Discussion

The discussion in this chapter has focused on one piece of legislation because of its importance not only in itself, but also in what it says about the formulation and implementation of social policies in Northern Ireland during the 1930s. The Mental Treatment Act (NI) 1932 brought to an end the use of nineteenth century lunacy laws, and formed the basis for the development of a mental health service based on assumptions related to illness and treatment. The impetus for reform came from England – from the work of the Macmillan Commission (HMSO 1926) the recommendations of which was reflected in the Mental Treatment Act 1930.

Everybody welcomed the new law, but it had not addressed the two major problems facing the asylums at the time – the presence in mental hospitals of children with a mental handicap and the acute shortage of money for any kind of development. Some argue that this law was a major breakthrough, that it transformed the world of lunacy, a hostile world peopled by 'inmates' and 'attendants' to one of illness, a caring world peopled by 'patients' and 'nurses'. It also removed the stigma from admission to a mental hospital, because people could seek treatment without fear of being certified as insane. Finally the Act was seen as the first step in the removal of judicial proceedings for admission to hospital.

Others argue that the 1932 Act was merely a cosmetic exercise, aimed at convincing the Westminster government that the laws in Northern Ireland were just as humane and as modern as those in Britain. The Act gave the appearance of progress because of changes in the mode of entry to institutions and in the labels applied to the world of mental disorder. However, because there was no change in the method of funding the asylums, there was little hope of progress in developing new services either attached to the hospital or based in a community or local area. Neither was there any possibility of real change in the daily lives of patients, some of whom would never return home because of the shame of having been institutionalized for a mental disorder. Even more damaging was the fact that any cosmetic exercise, by its nature, hides the real wound and prevents developments which might alter the nature of the situation. This is precisely what happened. Because it solved the major legal problems and provided a more acceptable language for the treatment of mental disorder, the Mental Treatment Treatment Act (NI) 1932 concealed serious deficiencies in the system.

3 A new mental health service – 1948

The establishment in July 1948 of a comprehensive health service structure marked the beginning of the most important period in this century for mental health policies in Northern Ireland. The Health Services Act 1948 made it the duty of the Ministry of Health and Local Government to promote 'services designed to secure improvement in the physical and mental health' of the people of the Province. (S.1) These services would be free of charge and would be available to all citizens. The Act authorized the establishment of two bodies to carry out the administration of the health services – the Northern Ireland General Health Services Board to take responsibility for personal medical services (provided by General Practitioners); and the Northern Ireland Hospitals Authority to take responsibility for all hospital and specialist services. (Part 2 & 3) One of the immediate effects of the Health Service Act (NI) was the integration of the mental hospitals into a general hospital structure, with all that implied in terms of financial and professional support.

The second important event, occurring simultaneously, was the passing of the Mental Health Act (NI) 1948. Although these two developments were interlinked, they represented different patterns of social policy formation. The establishment of a health care structure, centrally guided and funded, within which a coherent mental health policy could be articulated and implemented, was due primarily to a new commitment by the Westminster Government to public service provision in Northern Ireland. The enactment of a new mental health law abolishing judicial involvement in hospital admission procedures and establishing a Special Care Service (for people with a mental handicap), was primarily due to internal factors. The relatively stable situation within the Province, and the availability of money to support any initiatives, allowed for the development of a truly creative piece of legislation – the only mental health law in Northern Ireland with no parallel in Britain. There are two major questions to be answered about this period. What were the factors within Northern Ireland itself which shaped health policy developments during the post-war period and what difference did these developments make to mental health policy?

Post-war planning

> In the opinion of this house the Government of Northern Ireland ... is promoting the best interests of the people of Northern Ireland by adhering to its policy of maintaining social services in this part of the United Kingdom on the same standard as similar services are maintained in Great Britain. [PRO(NI) CAB 9C/48/1 : Draft motion 9 March 1943]

These sentiments were those of a Unionist government which disagreed with the highly interventionist policies of the Labour Government at Westminster. [PRO(NI) CAB 4/642/9] However, as Sir Basil Brooke (the new Prime Minister) realized, to have gone against the tide of post Beveridge policy reforms taking place in the United Kingdom would have been political suicide. Fortunately for Brooke, there was no serious organized opposition within the Northern Ireland Government to British policies for social service reforms and preparation for 'post-war reconstruction' paralleled that in Britain. One of the specialist committees set up to plan for new developments was the Select Committee on Health Services in Northern Ireland (1942-44). [HMSO(NI) 1944]

Northern Ireland had proved to be a valuable asset to Britain during the war, not only in practical terms (as a supplier of food, ships and manpower), but also because of its strategic position. This led to a change in the attitude of Westminster to the Province. Prime Minister Churchill made this clear many times. 'The bonds of affection between Great Britain and the people of Northern Ireland have been tempered by fire and are now, I firmly believe unbreakable.' (NIHC Deb. 4 May 1943, Vol. 26. Col. 466) Brooke was determined to take advantage of the positive British attitude and of the new financial climate, to raise the standard of public services. The debates spawned by the publication of the Beveridge Report (HMSO 1942) were followed with interest by Northern Ireland politicians (many of them new ministers appointed by Brooke). [PRO(NI) CAB 9C/48/1] Though aware that any public commitment to the extension of insurance and health schemes to Northern Ireland would require Treasury clearance, the Northern Ireland Cabinet was confident that the climate was right and that the Province would benefit equally from post-war developments in United Kingdom. [PRO(NI) CAB 4/513/7]

Discussions which took place in the early 1940s led to financial arrangements highly advantageous to Northern Ireland. It was the intention of both governments that from the middle of the 1940s parity of services and taxation between Great Britain and Northern Ireland would be the guiding principle of fiscal policy. (Ulster Year Book 1950, p. xxvii; Lawrence 1965, p. 77) Major Maynard Sinclair, Minister of Finance (NI), made this clear in his budget statement in May 1944.

> No definite statement can, however, be made until the British policy on social services generally has been finally determined. I need not remind the House that, whatever that policy may be, the adoption of all or any of the services popularly associated with the name of Beveridge will extend to Northern Ireland in accordance with the declared policy of your Government to ensure to our people the same social service amenities as exist in the rest of the United Kingdom. [NIHC Deb. 23 May 1944, Vol. 27. Col. 1252]

The Minister went on to assure the House that agreement had been reached that standards of essential public services would be equal in Northern Ireland and Great Britain. Because of the inadequate state of some of these services, this would entail extra expenditure before a basic level of acceptability could be reached. According to Sinclair this expenditure would be forthcoming.

> The existence of considerable leeway on these and other vital services having been recognized some considerable time ago, a general understanding has been reached with my Right Honourable Friend the Chancellor of the Exchequer, whereby means would be found to ensure equality of standards with the remainder of the United Kingdom. [NIHC Deb. 23 May 1944, Vol. 27, Col. 1258]

Though no definite estimate of cost had yet been decided, a preliminary review suggested that the amount required from the Northern Ireland Exchequer 'related solely to leeway (would) be in the neighbourhood of £6,000,000'. (Ibid. Col. 125)] 'Leeway' (the gap between the standard of service which actually existed and that which should exist) was one of the catchwords of the time. Together with the concept of 'parity' of services, it represented the political rhetoric with which the Stormont government wooed the Northern Ireland public. Standards varied between services and in many instances there was no clear idea of what they were being measured against. The vagueness of the measuring criteria made the political argument for extra finance stronger.

Changes in the financial relationship between Westminster and Stormont did not actually take place until 1948, but all plans being drawn up after 1944 were based on the principles outlined by the Minister of

Finance in May of that year. It was within this context that planning for health services development in Northern Ireland took place. There were three major influences on the plans which emerged; the Select Committee on Health Services in Northern Ireland 1942-44, the Northern Ireland Regional Hospitals Council 1942-48, and the Health Advisory Council for Northern Ireland 1944-48.

Planning for health

As in other parts of the United Kingdom, there was great optimism within Northern Ireland on what could be achieved with a centralized system of health and welfare. The task of planning for this great venture was approached with enthusiasm. The Select Committee on the Health Services (NI) which was appointed in December 1942 (the month the Beveridge Report was presented to the British Parliament) was the first to gather hard evidence on the poor state of the health services in the Province. [HMSO(NI) 1944] Concurrently with the work of the Select Committee was that of the Northern Ireland Regional Hospitals Council. The Select Committee, supported by the Hospitals Council, recommended the establishment of a new Ministry of Health, a Regional Hospitals Authority and a colony for mentally defective children. The rationale for a new Ministry of Health was clear. At the time, all of the six Ministries were involved in health services in some way.

> While the Ministry of Home Affairs might be called the public health authority for Northern Ireland, yet the Ministry of Labour administers the national health services, the Ministry of Education administers the school medical services, the Ministry of Agriculture administers the milk services and Diseases of Animals Acts, and the Ministry of Commerce administers the new Nursery Centres, while the Ministry of Finance exercises an over-riding authority as far as finance is concerned over all, and is responsible for compiling vital statistics. [HMSO(NI) 1944, para. 9]

A Ministry of Health and Local Government was set up in 1944, within a few months of the Committee's Report, taking over all of the health functions formerly held by other ministries. The major task facing it was planning for a ocmprehensive health and welfare system on a par with Britain. The Unionist government, though philosophically opposed to increasing state control over the lives of individual citizens, had accepted that the only way forward was to move with the tide of 'welfare state' ideology. [PRO(NI) CAB 4/642/9; Wichert 1991, p. 43]

As the 'appointed day' for the introduction of a comprehensive health service throughout the United Kingdom drew near, the Ministry had a number of well developed policy objectives. Most of these objectives, if achieved, would have a positive impact on mental health service development. These included the formation of a centralized hospitals authority to take responsibility for rate aided and voluntary hospitals, the provision of a high standard of treatment for all forms of illness including mental illness, the establishment of a Special Care Service to plan and provide services for those suffering from mental defect, and the targeting of specific areas of concern such as tuberculosis and mental illness for special service development.

Draft plans had already been drawn up by the Ministry, based on advice from the Health Advisory Council for Northern Ireland (1944-48), and from the Northern Ireland Regional Hospitals Council (1942-48). Both of these councils presented reports on different aspects of the health services. The Health Advisory Council carried out its work using specialist sub committees of people working in the area being studied. [For details of reports see HMSO(NI) 1948a, p. 2] The Regional Hospitals Council hased its recommendations on the findings of a comprehensive survey of hospitals funded by the Nuffield Foundation. [Regional Hospitals Council (NI) 1944 and 1946] Both of these Councils had subcommittees on mental health, and it was the specific work of these committees which guided policy formation and implementation in Northern Ireland during this period.

Northern Ireland Regional Hospitals Council The psychiatric subcommittee of the Council made recommendations very much in line with debates taking place in Britain. It argued for a central position for mental health within the general health service structure and for the extension of the role of psychiatry. [Regional Hospitals Council(NI) 1946, p. 65] In this it echoed the sentiments of the report of the Royal Medico Psychological Association on *The Future Organisation of Psychiatric Services*. (RMPA 1945)

The argument for the extension of psychiatry was first articulated in Northern Ireland by Dr Duncan Leys, one of the team who carried out the Hospitals Survey in 1943. Dr Leys had a more radical view than his fellow surveyors. He suggested that it was 'physical impossibility for first class work to be done under such conditions' as those which prevailed in mental hospitals in Northern Ireland. He was critical of the Province for having no laboratory technicians and no psychiatric research worker at mental hospitals, only one outpatient clinic, no attempt to treat the neuroses and no psychiatric advice for schools and law courts. His recommendations included the creation of an Institute of Psychiatry, with a Director holding a professorial appointment at the University; the enlargement of professional staff in mental hospitals in line with standards in general hospitals; and the establishment of a system of exchange for professional staff between general and mental hospitals. [Regional Hospitals Council (NI) 1944, para. 53. vi]

Health Advisory Council for Northern Ireland The work of the mental health services committee of the Health Advisory Council was quite different in character from that of the Hospitals Council. Its mandate extended beyond the boundaries of hospital provision. Two of its reports were of major importance – *Mental Deficiency in Northern Ireland* [HMSO(NI) 1946] and *Recommendations for change in the Mental Treatment Act (NI) 1932*. [PRO(NI) HSS 16/4/79] The former was the basis for the Special Care Service established in 1948, and the latter the basis for the Mental Health Act (NI) in the same year. The committee also made recommendations to the Ministry on other aspects of the mental health services, focusing in particular on the need to ensure that they did not become the 'cinderella' of the hospitals services in the new national health service structure. This could only be achieved by adequate representation by mental health practitioners on the proposed Northern Ireland Hospitals Authority, and the appointment of a committee (of the Authority) to guide mental health service development. [PRO(NI) HSS 16/3/104, Draft minute 10 on 27/6/1947]

It is clear from the Ministry papers of the time, that the recommendations of the Health Advisory Councils in general, and of this committee in particular were highly influential in guiding the direction of policy change during these formative years. [PRO(NI) HSS 16/3/104; HSS 16/4/79; HSS 16/2/26] The committee was successful in raising the profile of mental health issues, instrumental in ensuring a strong position for the mental hospitals within the structure of the Hospitals Authority (NIHA), and responsible for the major changes in the mental health law which took place in 1948. The influence of the committee continued after 1948, when seven of its members became the core group on the mental health services committee of the Northern Ireland Hospitals Authority. (NIHA 1951, p. 139) This was in stark contrast to the situation in England, where the Mental Health Standing Advisory Committee made very little impact on developments in the new NHS structure. (Webster 1991, p. 103)

Building the new service

When the 5th July 1948 arrived, hopes were high that post-war welfare state policies would have an immediate and positive effect on mental health services in Northern Ireland. The six psychiatrists who managed the mental hospitals were particularly optimistic about the emergence of psychiatry as a recognized specialty within medicine. However, the new policies could not be implemented easily within existing structures. To be successful, a number of radical changes had to be made in the legal basis for the services, in the overall administration of the hospitals, and in the way in which staff viewed themselves. The first wave of legal changes had already taken place in 1946, with the Public Health and Local Government (Administrative Provisions) Act (NI) and in the Public Health (Tuberculosis) Act (NI), the former establishing local health and welfare authorities and the latter the Northern Ireland Tuberculosis Authority (NITA). The second phase came in 1948, with the passing of the Health Services Act (NI) and the Mental Health Act (NI) which brought two new statutory bodies into being. General medical, pharmaceutical and dental schemes would in future be administered by the Northern Ireland General Health Services Board, and hospital services, including mental health and 'special care' (mental handicap), by the Hospitals Authority.

These developments were made possible by the existence of new financial agreements between the Chancellor of the British Exchequer and the Minister of Finance. The National Insurance Act (NI) 1946 guaranteed that insured persons in Northern Ireland would be entitled to the same benefits as their counterparts in Great Britain. This included cash payments for the unemployed, the sick, the retired, widows, orphans and women during maternity. (Lawrence 1965, p. 77) Further developments took the form of a social service agreement in 1949 (applying retrospectively to 5 July 1948), which covered national assistance, family allowances, non-contributory pensions and the health services. (Ulster Year Book 1950, p. xxxi)

Changing the law

The most radical changes in the mental health services came through special legislation – the Mental Health Act (NI) 1948. The first section of this Act set the tone. Its stated purpose was to 'provide a secure provision of services designed to improve and maintain the mental health of the people of Northern Ireland'. Because of the lack of any specific legislation in Northern Ireland on mental defect, it had been the original intention of the government to bring in a law similar to the English Mental Deficiency Acts of 1913 and 1927. However, the mental health services committee of the Health Advisory Council suggested a more radical option.

> We understand it is proposed, when the Health Services Bill has been considered by Parliament, that legislation to deal with mental defectives should be submitted. We would strongly urge that such an

opportunity should not be missed of bringing up to date the Lunacy and Mental Treatment Act 1821-1932, as cited in the Mental Treatment Act (NI) 1932, and introducing what we consider are necessary amendments and additions.

We would suggest to the Minister that the Act of 1932 and the preceding Lunacy Acts, in so far as they are still current after the passing of the Health Services Bill should be repealed by a Bill which would cover mental health, mental illness and mental deficiency in all their aspects. [PRO(NI) HSS 16/4/79, Recommendation 5]

The advice of the committee was taken and the legislation covered all aspects of mental health. The most important elements in the new Mental Health Act were: 1) The new emphasis on the promotion of mental health rather than the treatment of mental illness; 2) The total removal of judicial procedures (certification) from methods of admission to mental hospital (Part 2) ; 3) The inclusion of mental illness and mental defect in the same piece of legislation; and 4) The establishment of a separate Special Care Service to administer services for people with 'incomplete or arrested development of mind' (Part 3).

Admission procedures In future admission to a mental hospital would be on a voluntary or temporary basis. This meant that the need for certification by a judicial authority before admission was abolished. The 1932 Act had already introduced the idea of voluntary and temporary admissions which did not require judicial orders, though it was still possible to be certified as being 'of unsound mind' before admission. A significant number of patients continued to be admitted by means of certification, though the percentage had decreased from 85 per cent of total admissions in 1933 to 36 per cent in 1948. The following diagram illustrates the use of admission procedures since the passing of the Mental Treatment Act (NI) in 1932. Patients increasingly used voluntary admission procedures and by 1948 they constituted 41 per cent of total admissions. The period of most rapid change was between 1945 and 1948. Within an overall increase in admissions of 73 per cent, voluntary admissions increased by 160 per cent. The message of early treatment proclaimed by the Macmillan Commission (HMSO 1926) was being heard by the public.

The mental health services committee held the view that 'it was wrong for any patient to be admitted to a mental hospital as a certified patient with the accompanying stigma as such, where there was a reasonable prospect of recovery'. [HMSO(NI) 1946, Ss.6-7] Certification, however, did not disappear from the legislation completely, but remained as a safeguard on the liberty of the longstay patient.

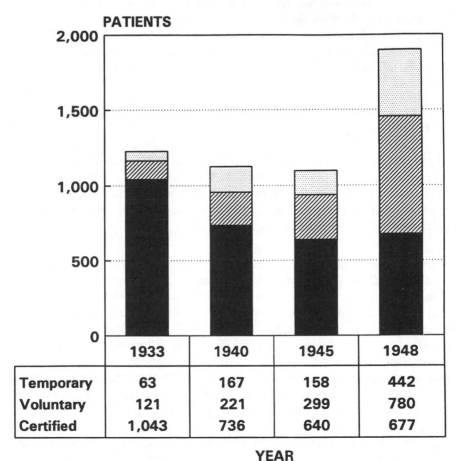

YEAR	1933	1940	1945	1948
Temporary	63	167	158	442
Voluntary	121	221	299	780
Certified	1,043	736	640	677

Figure 3.1   Mental hospital admissions for selected years 1933-48

Sources: *HMSO (NI) 1951; Weir 1949*

'When a temporary patient is judged by the Resident Medical Superintendent to have reached a stage where his recovery is improbable he may apply to "a judicial authority" to have the patient certified'. [Mental Health Act (NI) 1948, Sect. 9(1)] The fact that involvement by the judiciary in hospital treatment remained on the statute books was due to the specific intervention of the Lord Chief Justice during the preparation for the Act. The position was made clear to the mental health services committee by his representative on the committee, J. K. Davis, Legal Visitor in Lunacy and was articulated by the Minister of Health and Local Government in a speech prepared for the debate on the Bill in Parliament.

> The Government is strenuously opposed to any suggestion that prolonged detention in a mental hospital should be authorized by any method other than by order of a judicial authority. The Lord Chief Justice is also opposed to it.
> It is submitted that mental illness must be treated differently from physical illness inasmuch as mental illness involves detention against the will of the patient and in some instances against the wished of his friends or relatives. This means that the liberty of the subject is involved so that the problem is therefore more than a medical one and it is a fundamental principle of British justice that any such prolonged detention much be authorized only by a judicial authority. [PRO(NI) HSS 16/5/70]

The opposing argument, that of the medical profession, was put forward by Dr D. B. M. Lothian, Resident Medical Superintendent of the Downshire Hospital, and Vice Chairman of the committee, who argued that existing safeguards were sufficient. These included reports by the Resident Medical Superintendent (RMS) to the Ministry and the patient's right to communicate in writing to the Lord Chief Justice, the Governor of Northern Ireland or the Minister or to be visited by a Resident Magistrate.

> I understand that it is the liberty of the subject which is in question, and I recognize that this is fundamental, but in my opinion, it is attained by other statutory provisions . . . . These safeguards, and they will be reinforced if further recommendations of the Committee become law, appear to be ample in themselves, and to be much more effective than the submission of a medical certificate to a Justice of the Peace. [PRO(NI) HSS 16/4/79, Appendix to Recomm. 5]

Undoubtedly, Dr Lothian had the backing of many psychiatrists in Britain as well as in Northern Ireland, but the government was not yet ready to make the final move on this issue. There were two further changes made in admission procedures. The application for a temporary admission could be made (as before) by a relative or by a welfare officer, but in future it would have to be accompanied by only one medical certificate thus making it easier for people in rural areas to use this method of admission. This temporary order would admit a person 'who is suffering from mental illness and is unfit on account of his mental state to be received or to continue as a voluntary patient, or a person who is an addict.'[Mental Health Act (NI) 1948, S. 7(1)] The inclusion of addicts in the Act was due to the influence of the 1945 Mental Treatment Act in the Republic of Ireland. The mental health services committee had studied the Irish law and was particularly impressed by the decision to abolish judical proceedings from all aspects of mental hospital treatment. This was probably the last time that laws or services in the Republic were taken as a standard for judging similar laws and services in Northern Ireland, as after 1948 health services developed in different ways in the two parts of the country.

Other changes in the new Act included the introduction of protection for staff from unreasonable litigation. It also contained safeguards against wrongful detention – the obligation on the medical inspector to visit at least once per year, the right of the temporary or certified patient to request a visit from the resident magistrate, regulations concerning visiting committees and the duty of hospitals to display notices outlining patients' rights. These have all become standard practice in current mental health legislation but in 1948 they represented new ideas on rights to information as well as protection.

The other major change was the establishment of a Special Care Service for people with a mental defect. This had a significant effect on the mental health services after 1948, not only because of the development of separate services for this group of people, but also because it removed some of the confusion about mental illness and mental defect. A person requiring special care was defined in the Act as

> ... a person who has, in accordance with the provisions of this Act, been ascertained to be suffering from arrested or incomplete development of mind (whether arising from inherent causes or induced by disease or injury) which renders him socially inefficient to such an extent that he requires supervision, training or control in his own interests or in the public interest. [Mental Health Act (NI) 1948 S. 19(2)]

The decision to drop the terms 'mental defect' and 'mental sub-normality' had been taken on the recommendation of the mental health services committee. [HMSO(NI) 1946, para. 9] The implications of this part of the law (for the mental hospitals in particular) will be discussed in the next chapter. In spite of the fact that it did not go as far as some had hoped, the Mental Health Act (NI) 1948, by virtue of the language used and the changes in hospital admission procedures represented great progress. It was received with great acclaim in both Northern Ireland and Great Britain. The National Association for Mental Health (NAMH), in the August issue of its journal *Mental Health* praised the Act in the following terms.

> The Mental Health Act (NI) 1948 reflects a state of public opinion well in advance of that which has so far received legislative embodiment in this country, and is of special interest in that it surely outlines the shape of things to come. [Quoted in HMSO(NI) 1948b, p. 7]

Consequently, when it became law on 10 August 1948, it was introduced by the Ministry as 'a solid basis on which to build a mental health service for Northern Ireland which, in years to come, may well be an example to other countries'. [HMSO(NI) 1948b, p. 7] The Ministry warned, however, that legislation alone would not effect change.

> The Act ... is undoubtedly the foundation on which the future mental health service of Northern Ireland will be built, but however sound the foundation may be, the rest of the structure will need to be developed with equal care, otherwise strain and consequent weakness will be the inevitable result ... [HMSO(NI) 1948b, p. 7]

Northern Ireland had a long way to go before it could boast of having an adequate mental health service.

Changing the services

When the mental hospitals were transferred to the Northern Ireland Hospitals Authority in 1948, they were in a poor state of repair, outmoded in terms of basic sanitation and heating arrangements, overcrowded, uncomfortable and lacking in basic medical amenities such as laboratories, Xray equipment, and theatre facilities. (NIHA 1949, pp. 51-59) A number of improvements were planned as part of the overall development of hospital services in the Province. [HMSO(NI) 1951, p. 57; NIHA 1949, pp. 51-59] Beds in mental hospital beds amounted to 5,233 or 40 per cent of all hospital beds in Northern Ireland in 1948. The Ministry estimated that the province needed 6,700 additional beds, including 1,500 for mental hospitals and 1,000 in a colony for 'persons requiring special care'. [HMSO(NI) 1951, p. 75] The proposed expenditure on the provision of additional beds, essential improvements to outpatient departments, the building of new laboratories, and the provision of additional staff accommodation, over the period from 1949 to 1964, would be in the order of £12,000,000. It was expected that, by 1953, there would be 5,825 extra hospital beds in Northern Ireland, with 1,940 of these in hospitals or institutions for people suffering from mental illness or requiring special care. (Ibid)

As part of the modernization effort aimed at standarizing care in mental hospitals and integrating them with other hospitals in the Province, they were renamed. (See Appendix 2) The change of name served two different purposes – it confirmed psychiatric treatment as medical treatment and at the same time destigmatized the location of that treatment.

The staff Nurses constituted the largest staff group in mental hospitals. Though salaries and conditions of service had changed a number of times since the 1920s, the basic problem with regard to qualification had not. In 1948, in spite of incentives in some hospitals and sanctions in others, a significant number of nurses had received no formal training. [PRO(NI) HSS 16/4/26] Such was the chronic shortage of female nurses that, in order to attract employees from the Republic of Ireland, the Safeguarding of Employment Act (NI) 1947 was waived. It was by then accepted that mental nursing should have parity with general nursing, a parity which implied equal access to training.

> It is now generally accepted that the duties of the mental nurse are no less exacting than those of the general nurse and that understanding, training and intelligence to a high degree are required to make a successful career in the field of mental nursing. [HMSO(NI) 1948a, p. 66]

Before 1948 the process of professionalizing the nursing role was already under way. After the publication of the *Interim Report of the Select Committee on Health Services in Northern Ireland* [HMSO(NI) 1944], nurses' salary scales were standardized throughout Northern Ireland. This was a first step. The second was the replacement in 1948 of the certificate of the Royal Medico Psychological Association (RMPA) with that of the Registered Mental Nurse (RMN). (Donaldson 1983) In 1948 each of the six mental hospitals received provisional approval as a training school for the qualification of RMN, on the understanding that facilities and staffing levels would be improved to meet the requirements of the Joint Nursing and Midwives' Council for Northern Ireland. [HMSO(NI) 1951, p. 94]

During the same period social work and occupational therapy, were just beginning to make an appearance in Northern Ireland. In 1948 one psychiatric social worker was employed to look after members of HM forces 'discharged from service to psychiatric hospitals and neurosis centres' [HMSO(NI) 1948a, p. 64], and two worked in mental hospitals. [HMSO(NI) 1951, p. 91] It was virtually impossible to employ qualified occupational therapists and psychiatric social workers because of the lack of training courses for either profession within Northern Ireland itself.

Given the lack of qualified staff, it is hard to imagine how medical staff in mental hospitals could transform the service as planned by the Ministry. Medical and dental staff for the six mental hospitals totalled 28 in 1948. (NIHA 1954, p. 70) With no post-graduate training programme in either psychiatry or psychology in Northern Ireland, it was almost impossible to recruit qualified psychiatrists. The only solution, as far as the medical profession and the Ministry were concerned, was in line with the earlier recommendation of Dr Leys – the establishment of a chair of psychiatry at Queen's University Belfast. [Regional Hospitals Council (NI) 1944, para. 53] In 1948, therefore, when the standards from general hospital care were applied to mental hospitals there were glaring inadequacies at every level of the service. The most serious of these was probably not the badly equipped buildings or the austerity of the general physical environment in the hospitals, but the complete absence of a trained workforce to modernize the service as planned in this era of optimism.

The patients Who were the people for whom the new mental health services were being planned? In 1921 it had been relatively easy to define the target population of the lunacy services. It consisted of everyone registered as insane under the nineteenth century lunacy laws, regardless of their place of residence. Some were in district asylums, some in workhouses, and a relatively small number in private care and in the Central Criminal Lunatic Asylum, Dublin. By 1948 the situation had changed. The new mental health service had a broader mandate. Certainly it would still cater for seriously mentally ill people who needed hospital care but the assumption was that most of these illnesses would be treatable. It was clear in the post-war plans of the Ministry of Health and Local Government that acute care could only be improved if separated from chronic care. The difficulty with this model of care was that it did not fit the existing patient population of the mental health services.

In 1948 there were 5071 (3.8 per 1.000 population) patients in mental hospitals, and 235 'mentally afflicted' patients in workhouses in Northern Ireland. By this time there was no private care for mentally ill people, and 'criminal lunatics' were not listed separately because they were no longer treated separately. [HMSO(NI) 1951] As we have already seen in the last chapter, admission rates had been on the increase since 1921 (with the exception of the war years) and residency rates had followed the same pattern. This was in line with trends in both Britain (Jones 1972, p. 357) and the USA (Conrad and Schneider 1980, p. 62). The overall increase in the patient population between 1921 and 1948 was 27 per cent, with the two mental hospitals nearest Belfast (Northern Ireland's only large urban centre) have the highest rate of increase – Belfast Mental Hospital by 54 per cent and Antrim Mental Hospital by 33 per cent. The following chart illustrates the increase in patient numbers since 1921.

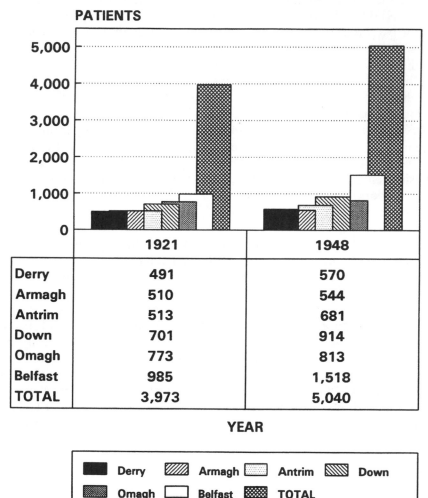

PATIENTS

	1921	1948
Derry	491	570
Armagh	510	544
Antrim	513	681
Down	701	914
Omagh	773	813
Belfast	985	1,518
TOTAL	3,973	5,040

YEAR

Derry Armagh Antrim Down Omagh Belfast TOTAL

Figure 3.2   Patients resident in mental hospitals 1921 and 1948

Source: HMSO (NI) 1924; HMSO (NI) 1951

Because there were no annual reports from the Ministry of Health and Local Government during the war years the amount of information available on patients during this period is very scant. The only details one can gather is on patients' age, legal status and mode of admission to hospital. The age of patients was discussed at great length because of the Ministry's concern with the increasing proportion of elderly patients being admitted which had implications for future services. Dr T. W. H. Weir, the new Senior Medical Officer (Mental Health), in an address to the Annual General Meeting of the Royal Medico Psychological Association, held in Dublin in 1948, told the meeting that an examination of the ages of patients on admission between 1943 and 1947 had shown that patients aged 65 years and upwards formed 21.5 per cent of total admissions.

> The great majority of these patients (were) suffering from permanent mental infirmity due to age or organic disease, where recovery was impossible and where nursing care rather than active psychiatric treatment was the requirement . . . (Weir 1949, p. 682)

He posed the rhetorical question : 'Should the mental hospital of the future, which is tending more and more to become an active treatment centre, be obliged to receive these old persons?' (Ibid) The Ministry reports gave more detail. Between 1945 and 1949 people over 65 years of age had constituted 21 per cent of admissions to mental hospitals, with 67 per cent of these suffering from dementia on admission. [HMSO(NI) 1951, p. 87] The increase in the numbers of elderly people being admitted to mental hospitals was not only due to the closure of workhouses in the Province but was part of the wider problem of the growing population of elderly patients in general hospitals and in the population at large. (Adams and Cheeseman 1951)

If the problem of the elderly in mental hospitals was causing concern the other area on which there is plenty of information during this period – mode of admission – was causing great optimism. The possibility of entering a public mental hospital on a voluntary basis had been introduced in 1932 and had been welcomed by the medical profession as long awaited progress. Admission statistics between 1932 and 1948 showed that the public also welcomed this new method of receiving treatment for mental disorders. In 1933, the first year of the operation of the new mental health law, certified patients formed 85 per cent of total admissions. By 1948 this had dropped to 36 per cent, with voluntary admissions now constituting 41 per cent of all admissions. (See Figure 3.1) Voluntary patients represented the new target population for the mental health service. These were people who were using the mental hospital just as they would use any other hospital – to have an illness treated and cured.

71

Planners hoped in the future to move chronic conditions out of the main stream of the new psychiatric service.

Discussion

Mental health policy in Northern Ireland during the 1920s and 1930s had been determined by the uncertainty of the political position in Northern Ireland, by the extreme financial restraint imposed by the Ministry of Finance on other ministries and by the pre-occupation of the new Unionist Government with issues of security. These factors had impeded any development in health and welfare services, although some changes in law, such as the Mental Treatment Act (NI) 1932, had occurred. By 1948, all of these factors had undergone significant change. The position of Northern Ireland within the United Kingdom was confirmed, civil unrest was not a pressing concern, and the financial restraints on social service spending had been withdrawn. The context was clearly conducive to a broadening of policy objectives and to an expansion of services.

Within this context, the actual changes in mental health policy, which took place in Northern Ireland, were the work of people within the Province itself. The Select Committee on Health Services in Northern Ireland 1942-44 laid the foundation for all later changes in health service structures. The Northern Ireland Regional Hospitals Council and the special Mental Health Services Committee of the Health Advisory Council worked out the detail of necessary changes in the law and in the structures of the mental health services. The resulting legislation, The Health Services Act (NI) 1948 and the Mental Health Act (NI) 1948, was comprehensive and, in the case of the latter, innovative.

Though influenced by debates in Great Britain, those working on the new policies for Northern Ireland were not constrained by them. They were also in tune with developments in the Republic of Ireland as was evident in the mental health legislation. This was probably the end of an era, as after 1948 social service provision in the two parts of Ireland diverged sharply and the grounds for cooperative or comparative work diminished. This reflected a deeper separation of identity between North and South, a separation which had been re-affirmed by differences in the war experience and strengthened by the financial commitment by Westminster to Northern Ireland in the post-war period. (See Wichert 1991, pp. 42-54) The next ten years would determine the direction and speed of growth in health, education and other social services. In spite of existing inadequacies, Northern Ireland politicians and civil servants hoped that with an injection of finance and the cooperation of the health professions, the mental health services would expand and develop in keeping with the most modern developments in the treatment of mental disorders.

4 Expansion and change – 1950s and 1960s

After fifty years of stagnation in mental service development, there followed two decades of unprecedented expansion. Integration of the mental hospitals into a general hospital structure meant an immediate increase in capital expenditure on buildings and equipment and a raising of standards in relation to staff numbers and qualification. However, the introduction of a comprehensive health care system brought its own problems. In England the cost of the NHS was causing grave concern, while in Northern Ireland the role of the powerful Northern Ireland Hospitals Authority became the subject of a Parliamentary Enquiry (Tanner Committee). During this period also, public unease (in England) about mental health legislation led to the appointment of a royal commission and further changes in the law throughout the United Kingdom.

Mental health service developments

There were two major strands to the developments which occurred in mental health services after 1948. The first was the redefinition of the territory covered by the services caused by the creation of a Special Care Service for people with a mental handicap. The second was the administrative relocation of mental hospitals within a general medical structure.

The Special Care Service

The presence of children in mental hospitals had been regarded as a scandal since the 1920s. Resident Medical Superintendents refused admission whenever possible but the hospitals were sometimes left with no option because of the lack of other facilities. The Mental Health Act (NI) 1948 provided the legal basis for the setting up of a separate service within the Hospitals Authority to develop a colony and other services (outside of the mental hospitals) for people with a mental handicap. Developments were slower that anticipated and in 1950 the Secretary of the Hospitals Authority E. H. Jones, wrote to the Ministry about the seriousness of the situation. With the exception of Muckamore, Co. Antrim (with 17 beds) there were no suitable special care beds in Northern Ireland. He estimated that there were approximately 100 people of 'lower grade type' in welfare hostels, with 22 children in Belfast City Hospital. In addition, there were 31 'high grade' girls who required institutional care with approximately 15 of these in mental hospitals. Some of these girls had their illegitimate babies with them. [PRO(NI) HSS 16/5/150, letter of 11/2/1950]

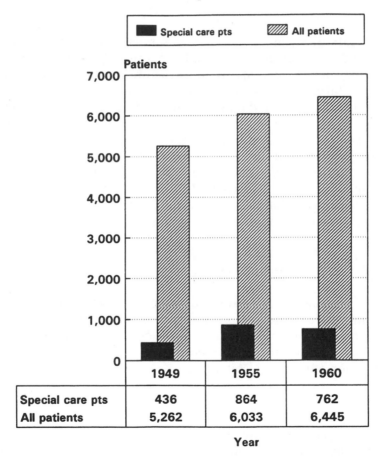

Figure 4.1   Special care patients in mental hospitals 1949-60

Source: HMSO (NI) 1951; NIHA 1955 & 1960

In addition to children, there were a number of adults with a mental handicap in mental hospitals. From 1948 onward each hospital kept a record of these patients. In 1949 the number was 436 (eight per cent of the resident patient population). In 1950 the official figure had increased to 615 (12 per cent of the resident patient population). [HMSO(NI) 1952, p. 35] This increase was probably due to the reclassification of existing patients rather than to any increase in admissions as management committees and medical staff in mental hospitals in 1949 hoped to transfer these patients to Special Care Service accommodation in the near future. However, as can be seen from Figure 4.1, the situation had not changed very much by 1960. The number of special care patients in mental hospitals was still significant in that year, constituting 12 per cent of the total patient population.

What had changed was the pattern of admission. By 1960 mental hospitals were not admitting patients with a mental handicap. This major change was due to the Hospitals Authority decision to make provision for special care patients in the community (who required hospital care), before transferring patients from mental hospitals. (Mulligan et al. 1964, p. 8) This led to the expansion of residential facilities at Muckamore Abbey, Co. Antrim, and Tower Hill, Co. Armagh, and the development of four other smaller hostels. (NIHA 1960, p. 159) In spite of these developments mental hospitals still constituted 41 per cent of the special care residential accommodation in 1960. (See Appendix 3)

The first decade of the Special Care Service had made little impact on either the patient population or staffing levels in mental hospitals. However, the establishment of the service had brought about an important change in attitude. The distinction between mental illness and mental handicap and the need to provide different services to meet the needs of each group, were now accepted by the public as well as by professionals. By highlighting this distinction the Special Care Service had put new boundaries around services for mentally ill people.

Hospital expansion

The task facing the Hospitals Authority was immense. Early reports referred frequently to the inadequacy of existing services and the need for new buildings, new equipment and increased professional training opportunities for staff. (NIHA 1948-53) The Mental Health Services Committee, which was the channel through which all policy decisions about mental health were made during the twenty five year lifespan of the Hospitals Authority, was clear in its evaluation of the situation.

    . . . existing mental hospitals services were inadequate to provide for
    all the mentally ill persons in Northern Ireland requiring hospital

treatment and preliminary consideration was given to extensions to the existing hospitals and also to the building of a new hospital at Gransha, Londonderry . . . (NIHA 1950, p. 20)

In the first year of its existence, the Hospitals Authority set out to improve and supplement accommodation at all mental hospitals. A two pronged programme was initiated to bring about the necessary changes.

Under the first part of the programme, major schemes of renovation and modernization are being carried out to bring the existing mental hospital buildings into line with accepted present day standards. Under the second part of the programme, new buildings are being erected and brought into use as quickly as possible, thus providing the additional beds so badly needed to relieve overcrowding. [HMSO(NI) 1956, p. 27]

Improvements included the upgrading of existing kitchens, laundries and bathrooms, the adaptation of treatment areas to provide proper laboratory, occupational therapy and Xray departments, and the provision of new furnishings and equipment. New buildings included additional wards, new residences for nursing and medical staff, and new treatment facilities. By 1955, new buildings had been erected at all six mental hospitals bringing 310 beds (of the planned 1,500) into use. [HMSO(NI) 1956, p. 27] At five of the hospitals the new buildings were dual purpose, which meant they could be converted into casualty or general hospital purposes if the need arose. By 1958, the first stage of the new mental hospital at Gransha, Derry, was completed – this represented an additional 178 beds. [HMSO(NI) 1959, p. 25] The planned 1,000 bed colony for 'special care' (mental handicap) patients did not materialize as quickly as envizaged, but by the end of 1960 there were 600 patients living in the new colony at Muckamore Abbey, Co. Antrim. (NIHA 1961, p. 66) In 1961 both Purdysburn Hospital and Downshire Hospital had new Nurses Homes, the administrative building and recreation hall were completed at Gransha and extensive modernization of patient accommodation had taken place at the Tyrone and Fermanagh Hospital and at Purdysburn Hospital. (NIHA 1960, p. 65 and 1961, p. 69)

The result was a raising of the living standards and of the quality of general medical care and treatment. During the 1950s treatments such as ECT, insulin treatment and prefrontal leucotomy were being used on patients from all mental hospitals, although leucotomies were performed only at Purdysburn Hospital because of the need for special theatre equipment. By the 1960s the treatment regime had changed due to the availability of psychotropic drugs and to critical scrutiny of earlier treatments. Insulin treatment had been abandoned completely and leucotomy, which had been under review since the publication in 1947 of the English Board of Control research, was strictly controlled. [PRO(NI) HSS 16/3/125; See also Jones 1972, p. 29; Conrad and Schneider 1980, p. 61] With improved access to treatment and an increase in hospital beds, came a steady growth in patient numbers. As the following chart shows, admission rates rose more quickly than discharge rates, causing this upward trend.

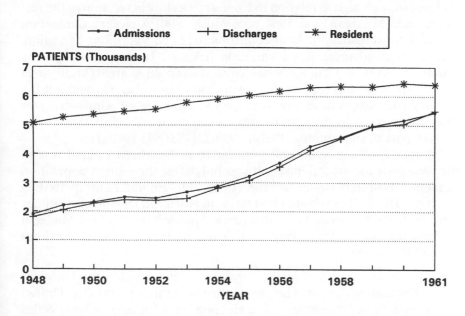

Figure 4.2 Admissions and discharges to mental hospitals 1948-61

Source: Min. Health and Loc Gov (NI)

Throughout the United Kingdom during the 1950s, increased numbers of beds and of attendances at outpatients clinics were taken as indicators of an improved service. In Northern Ireland available beds rose from 5,071 in 1948 to 6,486 in 1961. (See Appendix 1) This represented 3.8 per 1,000 of the population in 1948 and 4.5 per 1,000 in 1961. When the 1961 figure is compared to that of England, which was 3.3 per 1,000, and that of the Republic of Ireland, which was 7 per 1,000, it is clear that Northern Ireland, though high in relation to England was low in relation to the rest of Ireland. (Mulligan et al. 1964, p. 5; Walsh 1990) A closer examination of the 1961 statistics for both countries revealed variations by region. Within England there was a variation from 2.3 beds per 1,000 in the Sheffield region to 7.2 in the South West Metropolitan area. (Mulligan et al. 1964, p. 5) Within Ireland there were variations also. Throughout the country, rural areas have always tended to have higher admission rates than urban areas, as do western areas when compared with areas in the eastern part of the country. [Walsh 1990; DHSS(NI) 1990a)

Prior to 1960 the main policy initiative in Northern Ireland was to increase beds for mental illness. It was only after the patient population in mental hospitals began to drop (in 1959 in England and in 1961 in Northern Ireland) that higher bed ratios in Northern Ireland came under scrutiny. In the survey of psychiatric services, undertaken by Dr J. Mulligan in 1964, the idea of applying British norms to services in Northern Ireland was rejected.

> This is one branch of medicine where no justification can be found for accepting figures of bed requirement of other parts of the United Kingdom as a standard . . . The Hospital Plan for England and Wales is not applicable to Northern Ireland because so many condition are different. (Mulligan et al. 1964, p. 5)

The authors were referring to the statement in the Hospital Plan (HMSO 1962) which predicted that by 1975 the bed requirement within the United Kingdom would be 1.8 beds per 1,000 population for mental illness. Mulligan suggested a norm for Northern Ireland of between 3.28 and 3.64 per 1,000 which was a reduction of approximately one bed per 1,000 on the 1961 figure. (Mulligan et al. 1964, p. 7)

In contrast to the discussion on bed rates, the continuing increase in outpatient numbers was welcomed by all. The statistics are difficult to interpret because the numbers refer to attendances rather than to numbers of patients. However, it is evident that the outpatient clinic, almost non existent in 1948, had become a valuable part of the treatment for mental illness by the early 1960s. During this period, all of the outpatient clinics were staffed from the mental hospitals though some were held in general hospitals. Purdysburn clinics, for example, continued to be held at the Royal Victoria Hospital, Belfast. The following diagram illustrates the dramatic development of this method of treatment.

Mentally Ill Out-Patients

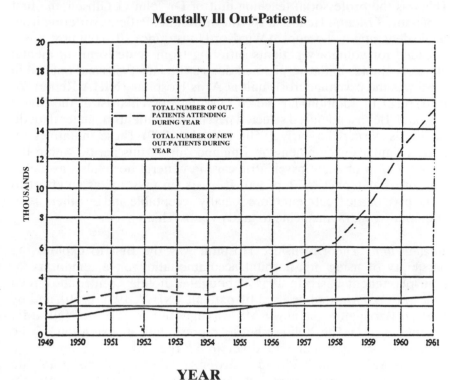

YEAR

Figure 4.3   Psychiatric outpatient attendances 1949-61

Source: HMSO (NI) 1962, p.10

The increases in both outpatient attendances and in bed numbers were a reflection of both increased supply (commitment of financial resources) and increased demand (willingness of people to use the services). In the eyes of the public the mental health services had indeed been transformed between 1948 and 1960 – from being a system of containment to one providing care and treatment.

New schemes

Three important developments were initiated from the mental hospitals but not confined to them : psychiatric units in general hospitals; satellite units attached to mental hospitals ; and day hospital treatment.

79

Psychiatric units in general hospitals Windsor House (at Belfast City Hospital), officially opened in 1960, was the first of these new units. This was the professorial teaching unit of Dr John G. Gibson, the first Professor of Mental Health in Northern Ireland. Patients suffering from senile dementia had occupied Windsor House since 1926 but now it was intended for voluntary patients suffering from acute forms of mental illness. A similar initiative planned during the late 1950s and opened in 1961, was the psychoneurosis unit at Ards Hospital. (NIHA Report for 1961, p.12) In addition, Dr Pierce O'Malley, psychiatrist at the Mater Hospital, Belfast admitted selected psychiatric patients to general medical wards during the early 1950s. (Wright 1989) These initiatives reflected similar developments in England during this period where the incorporation of acute psychiatric care in general hospitals was highly controversial. (Jones 1972, p. 300) It was seen by some as an effort to make psychiatric treatment more socially acceptable and by others as an attempt by general medicine to take over psychiatry.

Satellite units The Downshire Hospital was the first to explore the possibility of using non-hospital accommodation on a temporary or semi permanent basis. In 1954 it bought a holiday centre at Tyrella beach in Co. Down, to be used by patients (NIHA 1957, p. 60), and by 1961 Dr Berrington, the new RMS, was agitating for a hostel. (NIAMH Minutes 8/5/61) The holiday house represented an extension of the theme of occupational and diversional therapy for patients. The mental hospital, which already encompassed the patients' total life experience, was now providing extensive social and recreational facilities. By extending this to holiday arrangements, a safe happy alternate world was being constructed for the longstay patient population. Literature on the negative effects of institutionalization had not yet reached Northern Ireland.

The opening of the holiday home at Tyrella was described in terms of a 'therapeutic community' (a concept made famous by Dr Maxwell Jones at Belmont and Dingleton in England). (Jones 1968)

> In order to . . . encourage initiative and stimulate interest, attention has been concentrated on those projects offering hope of good development. Patients are being encouraged to do things for themselves and by themselves, consequently much of the work on the new holiday home at Tyrella and a great deal of work at the hospital has been carried out by the patients . . . The hospital is pursuing its ideal of the therapeutic community, using occupational therapy not as a means of passing time, but as a way to individual development and as a means of contributing to community life and at the same

time establishing more and stronger links with what used to be thought of as 'the world outside'. (NIHA 1957, p. 35)

As a method of treatment for mental illness, the 'therapeutic community' was quickly replaced by that of community care, which shifted the focus from life within the hospital to the possibility of life in the community.

Day hospitals Discussions on plans for opening a day hospital in Belfast, with links to Holywell Hospital, Antrim, began in the mid 1950s. This was intended for selected patients 'especially those suffering from neurotic complaints'. (NIHA 1954, p. 61) Premises were purchased in 1959 and the first day hospital in Northern Ireland opened at Cliften Street, Belfast in August 1961. (NIHA 1959, p. 67)

> At the end of the year this new service, the first of its kind in Northern Ireland, was being fully used by general practitioners and the mental hospitals. The number of admissions during this period was 112 and total attendances at the three outpatient clinics held in conjunction with the Day Hospital were 74. In addition to these facilities, a successful social club was being held weekly for the benefit of expatients and their relatives, and the attendance at the Club meetings was approximately 30/40 each evening. (NIHA 1961, p. 31)

For the first time it was possible to receive daily treatment for a mental disorder without being hospitalized in the traditional sense of the word. Critics would say that, in spite of these initiatives, nothing much had changed in some of the back wards of the mental hospitals – the wards which were peopled by longstay chronic patients and unqualified staff inherited from the pre 1948 era. The main obstacle to progress was not the lack of finance but the lack of qualified staff.

Professional developments

The new service called for the employment of doctors trained in psychiatry, psychiatric social workers, nurses with qualifications in psychiatry, occupational therapists and clinical psychologists. Within Northern Ireland the pool of potential staff was small and until the late 1950s there were no opportunities for specialist training in the Province. In medicine the situation did not change significantly until after the appointment, in 1957, of John G. Gibson as the first Professor of Mental Health at Queen's University. However, the actual numbers of doctors working in mental hospitals in 1960 was more than double the number in 1948. The following table shows the staffing for both years.

Table 4.1
Staffing in mental hospitals in Northern Ireland for 1948 and 1960
(approved establishments)

Establishment	July 1948	December 1960
Consultants	12	22
Other Medical staff	13	46
Special Depts.	10	55
Nurses	976	1,538
Admin. & Clerical	38	96
Chaplains	26	27
Maintenance	79	151
Farms & Gardens	72	75
Domestic & General	290	536
TOTAL	1,516	2,546

Source: NIHA Report for 1960, p. 65.

The statistics for medical staff in mental hospitals in 1960 in the context of overall hospital provision gives an indication of the relative understaffing in psychiatry. Out of a total of 329 consultants and specialists employed by the Hospitals Authority, 29 were psychiatrists. (NIHA 1960, p. 72) In addition, out of a total of 258 non-consultant medical staff employed by the Authority, 42 were working in mental hospitals or in the new Department of Mental Health at Queen's University (Special Care Service excluded). This was in the context of a total bed complement for all hospitals of 17,129 of which 6,445 (38 per cent) were in the six mental hospitals. (NIHA 1960, pp. 74 and 132) It could be argued that a fair distribution of medical staff would have been 125 for consultants and specialists and 98 for non-consultant staff (38 per cent).

Nursing as a profession continued to gain status after 1948, as standards of entry to training became more strict and as salaries and conditions of service improved. However, in spite of efforts on the part of the Joint Nursing and Midwives Council for Northern Ireland to bring training for mental health care into line with general health care, professional standards were different. Difficulties in recruiting female staff led to the introduction in 1956 of the lower grade of State Enrolled Assistant Nurse. [HMSO(NI) 1957b, p. 28] This eased the situation but did not improve the image of the mental nurse.

The emergence of the newer mental health professionals – psychiatric social workers, psychologists and occupational therapists – was a significant development in mental hospitals in England during the 1950s. This was not the case in Northern Ireland. Training for psychiatric social work did not begin at Queen's University, Belfast until the end of the 1950s. Secondment arrangments to British courses resulted in only ten and a half full time posts being filled by 1957. [HMSO(NI) 1958, para. 20] Although all mental hospitals had occupational therapy departments since the early 1940s, training did not begin in Northern Ireland until 1961. (NIHA 1961, p. 17) Before this, departments were staffed by nurses with a special interest in occupational therapy.

Clearly the commitment to upgrading mental health services was being slowed by the lack of properly qualified staff. This applied to nursing, medicine, occupational therapy and social work. In spite of 'generous secondment arrangements' by the Hospitals Authority, recruitment to specialist positions, which required a period of training outside of Northern Ireland, was not successful. Professional organizations, such as the British Medical Association, the Royal College of Psychiatry, the Royal College of Nursing and the Association of Psychiatric Social Work, lobbied for the establishment of academic training courses and research facilities in the Province, convinced that this constituted the only road to professional progress. The establishment of professional training courses was not a simple matter, because of the cost implications. By the mid 1950s everyone was fuly aware of the huge financial investment involved in providing a comprehensive health servic3e. Before looking at the other major development in relation to mental health policy in Northern Ireland during this period [the Mental Health Act (NI) 1961], it is useful to discuss briefly the two problems which had arisen in the general health services structure at the time. The first was the growing cost of the services and the second increasing discontent with the Hospitals Authority.

Financial and administrative problems

The cost of the health services was one of the major concerns in relation to the NHS throughout the United Kingdom during the early 1950s. Within the first few months of its introduction, it became obvious that projected estimates had been too low. As a result, the government voted a supplementary estimate of £59 million for 1948-49 and one of £98 million for 1949-50. (Klein 1983, p. 34) Rising costs were due to the increased demand for services, a rise in the cost of living in the immediate post-war period and the unacceptably low level of health care provision in some areas prior to 1948. In an effort to stem the rising tide in demand and to generate income, a prescription charge of one shilling was introduced in Great Britain in 1949 and in Northern Ireland in 1950. Charges were extended to dentures and glasses in 1951. [HMSO(NI) 1952, p. 6: HMSO(NI) 1954, p. 22] The introduction of health charges within the newly created 'welfare state' structure not only precipitated the resignation of Aneurin Bevan, but also aroused such controversy that a Parliamentary Committee (Guillebaud) on the cost of the NHS was appointed.

The Guillebaud Committee (1953-56) argued that many of the accusations of extravagance which had been levelled at the health services were unfounded and that high costs were due to initial expenses in setting up a comprehensive health service and to the poor state of the nation's health prior to 1948. Both of these factors were temporary and expenses were expected to decrease in future. Guillebaud also pointed out that in spite of the growth in public expenditure on the NHS since 1948, the cost as a percentage of the gross national product had actually fallen in the period from 1948 to 1954. (HMSO 1956, para. 61) In an effort to parallel some of the work of the Guillebaud Committee, the Ministry of Health and Local Government invited Professor Brian Abel-Smith (one of the committee's chief advisers) to compare health service costs in Northern Ireland with those in England and Wales for the period 1949 to 1956. Abel-Smith found that current costs of health services per head of population were consistently lower in Northern Ireland than in England and Wales. In 1956 this was £11.1s. in England and Wales and £9.12s. in Northern Ireland. Capital investment on the contrary, escalated from over twice as much in 1949/50 to four times as much in 1955/56. In 1955/56 capital investment per head was 24 shillings (£2) in Northern Ireland as against six shillings in England and Wales.

Planned capital expenditure on hospitals for the first 15 years after the establishment of the Hospitals Authority (1949-64) was of the order of £12 million. [HMSO(NI) 1951, p. 75] Not all of the expenditure was to provide additional beds, so it is difficult to estimate how much of this was targeted towards mental health services. However, on the basis of the number of planned beds (8,500 in all including 2,500 mental health and mental handicap) it can be estimated that approximately 29 per cent of the £12 million was intended for mental health and mental handicap services. As it transpired, costs were much higher than anticipated. Between July 1948 and December 1953, the Hospitals Authority's capital expenditure amounted to £4,250,000. During the same period in England and Wales (with a population exceeding 30 times that of Northern Ireland) capital expenditure on hospitals was £45 million. [HMSO(NI) 1955, para. 51] In the light of escalating costs, plans for expansion were rigorously reviewed during the mid 1950s. (NIHA Reports 1953-55) Neverthless, as Abel-Smith demonstrated, there was a substantial commitment to capital investment in the hospital sector in Northern Ireland prior to and including 1956.

Unfortunately, the impact of the investment was not immediately apparent. Because of the delays in carrying out what were regarded as necessary structural improvements in hospitals throughout the Province, serious discontent at the bureaucracy of the Hospitals Authority was expressed as early as 1952. Annual reports from mental hospitals, which had been full of optimism in 1949, were soon peppered by complaints about the slow pace of improvement. The Downshire Hospital management committee in its third report, made its dissatisfaction clear.

> Our work has again been hampered by the shortage of accommodation in every department of the hospital and despite the admissions on the part of all deputations from the Authority that our need in this respect is urgent, we still have not had one bed added since 1948, nor an additional square inch to the appallingly small space in which the secretary's department has to carry out its duties . . . (Downshire 1952, p. 1)

In the same year there were complaints from other hospitals about the centralization of decision making in the Hospitals Authority.

The management committee of Holywell Hospital, Antrim wrote:

> . . . the service generally would benefit also by a measure of devolution in respect of capital expenditure, developments which would enable projects approved within certain expenditure limits to be dealt with directly by the management committee concerned instead of by headquarters staff. (Holywell 1952, p. 12)

As these complaints became widespread, local politicians became involved in the debate. They broadened the issue and raised fundamental questions about the apparent lack of electoral control over the Hospitals Authority and the growing power of administrators within what was seen as an increasingly bureaucratic organization unresponsive to public need.

The role of the Hospitals Authority The establishment of independent organizations such as the Hospitals Authority and the General Health Services Board (NI) to coordinate and plan services, was seen by the Ministry as the only way of standardizing care throughout the Province. Local needs could, it was felt, be communicated to these organizations through hospital management committees and local professional committees. [NIHA 1950, pp. 21-35: HMSO(NI) 1951, pp. 44-48] However, communication channels were not successfully established, as was clearly demonstrated by the two enquiries on health services in Northern

Ireland which took place during this period. The first enquiry, one internal to the Hospitals Authority, was carried out by the Corbett Committee between April and October 1954. (NIHA 1954b) The second, a Parliamentary enquiry, took place between June 1954 and April 1955. [Tanner Report, HMSO(NI) 1955b]

Though precipitated by the same events, the two enquiries focused on different issues. The major theme, dominating discussion in both, was the excessive power being wielded by the Hospitals Authority. Particularly irksome to hospital management committees was the fact that decisions on capital expenditure on equipment in excess of £25 had to be made at headquarter level [HMSO(NI) 1955b, para. 137] and all decisions had to be debated in one of the numerous specialist committees of the Hospitals Authority before being passed to the Planning and General Purposes Committee for approval. This led to delays in decision making – delays which were seen by hospital management committees as the unecessary trappings of bureaucracy. (NIHA 1954b, p. 25) According to the Corbett Committee :

> A major criticism of the Authority, and one for which there is more justification than other criticism to which they are subjected, is that there is undue delay in reaching decisions and in communicating them to the persons and bodies concerned. (NIHA 1954b, p. 25)

Stronger sentiments were expressed by the Tanner Committee in its report.

> Many complaints were made to us of delays on the Authority's part in giving decisions, of arbitrary behaviour by the Authority and of crippling restrictions on the powers of decision of management committees. [HMSO(NI) 1955b, para. 131]

It was suggested that the Hospitals Authority should be abolished, or at least stripped of its executive functions and turned into an advisory body. Other suggestions were full of contradictions. For example, there were demands for greater ministerial and Parliamentary control over the hospital services alongside demands for greater freedom and autonomy for local hospital management committees. The Tanner Committee recommended a change in the relationship between the Hospitals Authority and the Ministry of Health and Local Government to ensure more Parliamentary control – the 'Authority should be placed in the relation to the Ministry of an agent to a principal'. (Ibid. para. 96) This would mean adopting a structure akin to that of the Regional Hospitals Boards in England and Wales, with the Hospitals Authority acting on behalf of the Ministry rather than as an independent body.

As a result of the Guillebaud Committee in Great Britain and of the

Tanner and Corbett committees in Northern Ireland, a number of changes were made in the financing of all hospitals. From the beginning of April 1954, each hospital was given a block allocation to be used at the discretion of the management committee. All expenditure in that year would have to be met from this money with the exception of increases in salaries and wages. Approval for the appointment of additional medical and senior staff would still have to be sought from the Hospitals Authority. However, committees could appoint additional junior staff without seeking prior approval provided they had sufficient funds to do so. (NIHA 1955, p. 14) For the next decade, hospital committees used their autonomy to capitalize on a situation of increased public expenditure and relative peace. (Simpson 1983, p. 93; Darby 1983, p. 23) Those involved in service delivery were able to devote their energy to improving standards of care and treatment. For people suffering from a mental illness it was a time of great hope, engendered not only by the availibity of new treatments but also by further changes in the law which made these treatments more accessible.

Mental Health Act (NI) 1961

Changes in mental health legislation in England and Wales in 1959 meant that the existing law in Northern Ireland [Mental Health Act (NI) 1948], which had been regarded as progressive at the time, was now out of date. The work of the Royal Commission on Mental Illness and Mental Deficiency 1954-57 (Percy Commission) was followed with keen interest by civil servants in the Ministry and by members of the Mental Health Services Committee of the Hospitals Authority, as it was inevitable that it would have an impact here.

The preparatory phase

Preparation for changes in the law took the form of consultations between the Ministry and interested bodies such as the Mental Health Services Committee of the Hospitals Authority, the newly formed Northern Ireland Association for Mental Health (NIAMH) and local branches of professional organizations such as the British Medical Association and the Association of Psychiatric Social Work. Discussion centred on issues raised by the Percy Commission, the content of the English Mental Health Act 1959 and problems specific to Northern Ireland arising out of the implementation of the Mental Health Act (NI) 1948. The foundation for the new Northern Ireland Act had been laid in England, not only in the work of the Percy Commission but also in the two social work reports published in the 1950s – the Mackintosh Report (HMSO 1951) and the Younghusband Report (HMSO 1959) and in the public education campaign of the National Association for Mental Health.

The message of the Percy Commission was clear. The right to treatment rather than the need for protection would dominate the new era of mental health legislation.

> We recommend that the law should be altered so that whenever possible suitable care may be provided for mentally disordered patients with no more restriction of liberty or legal formality than is applied to people who need care because of other types of illness, disability or social difficultry. Compulsory powers should be used in future only when they are are positively necessary to override the patients's own unwillingness or the unwillingness of his relatives, for the patient's own welfare or for the protection of others. (HMSO 1957, para. 70)

This was quite a change from the position adopted by the government in Northern Ireland during the preparation for the Mental Health Act (NI) 1948 when psychiatrists unsuccessfully lobbied for the removal of all judicial procedures in admissions. [PRO(NI) HSS 16/5/70; HSS 16/4/79] The change was due to the acceptance by the Percy Commission of a new model of care for mental illness. (Unsworth 1987) For the first time since the establishment of an asylum system in the early nineteenth century, there was a radical shift of focus to community based services as a method of treatment. The shift towards a model of service provision in which the mental hospital was peripheral rather than central, began in Britian and America almost simultaneously. (Conrad and Schneider 1980, p. 66: Jones 1988, p. 7) In Northern Ireland the focus was still on improving life within mental hospitals and there was no pressure for legal change. However, it was incvitable that the law would change in line with Britain. No special preparatory committee was set up in Northern Ireland probably due to the fact that there was no opposition to any of the principles underlying the 1959 English Mental Health Act.

Issues and debates The new legislation was formulated in record time. Having being introduced to the House of Commons of the Northern Ireland Parliament on 24 April 1961, it was passed to the Senate on 28 June and received Royal Assent on 19 December. (NIHC Deb. 1961, Col. 1411; NI Sen Deb. 1961, Col. 515) In principle it differed little from the Mental Health Act (NI) 1948, but there were a number of important changes arising from new perspectives which had emerged in the intervening twelve years. The designation of the mental hospital as the only type of hospital within which treatment could be received was no longer seen as necessary. In future patients could be admitted to any hospital. [Mental Health Act (NI) 1961, Sect. 6] The purpose of this section was clear. Psychiatric care had to be divorced from treatment in a mental hospital. Admission would be on the same basis as for physical illness – if hospital care was judged necessary by the doctor and the patient was willing to accept then he or she would be admitted. For patients not willing to accept hospitalization, the formal procedure (temporary admission) introduced in 1948, was changed slightly. The application for admission could be made by a relative or a designated welfare officer and would only require one medical certificate. (Sect. 12-18)

The reaction against legalism, already apparent in the legislation of the 1930s and 1940s, was even stronger in the new Act. The power of the medical profession was enhanced not only by the new admission procedures, but also by the removal of the judicial authority from decisions about long term compulsory hospitalization. In future, the hospital management committee could authorize continuing care and/or treatment based on a medical recommendation. (Sect. 32) The arguments which had been advanced in 1948 on the need to safeguard the liberty of the individual were no longer seen as relevant in the more enlightened environment of the 1960s. The battle which took place in England prior to the 1959 Act between those who favoured more legal safeguards and those who opposed them has been well documented by both Jones (1972) and Unsworth (1987). In Northern Ireland the battle had already been won in 1948 by the anti-legal lobby. Medical control over compulsory hospitalization was now granted completely. In order to protect patients against any possible abuse of medical power, there would be a Mental Health Review Tribunal for Northern Ireland. (Part. V1) Members would be appointed from three groups – medical, legal and lay – and would normally consist of three members (one from each panel) during a sitting. The task of the Tribunal would be to examine the case of any patient being held in hospital on a compulsory basis.

In contrast to its English counterpart, the Northern Ireland Bill proposed no extra powers or funding to local welfare authorities to develop community services. This omission was criticized by two Members of Parliament as the draft legislation passed through the Northern Ireland Parliament. Desmond Boal, a leading Belfast barrister and MP for Shankill, voiced his criticisms during the debate on the Second Reading. 'I believe community services are being neglected. They are, I regret to say, not mentioned in this Bill and they ought to be.' (NIHC Deb. 1961, Col. 2073) Boal suggested that at least permissive powers should be given to local welfare authorities, and at most mandatory powers and central funding. Senator Marion Greeves also expressed her concern.

It has been stated that within a decade all the county mental hospitals will be closed. This disclosure of the future policy of the Hospitals Authority fills me with alarm and apprehension ... Many (patients) have been in institutions for a lifetime and have become accustomed to the care, protection and security which the hospitals offer. Are they to be thrown out into a world of which they know little or nothing – unknown strangers from another era, often unwanted by relatives who in some cases have abandoned them. These unfortunate people cannot be forced to live with relatives who do not want them. In the last resort they will be thrust on the welfare authorities, which will have to build new and expensive homes at great expense to the country. (NI Sen. Deb. 1961, Cols. 794-795)

Senator Greeves urged the government to make increased grants available to welfare committees to cover this heavy expenditure and remove 'an unfair burden from the already heavily taxed ratepayer'. (Ibid. Col. 620) Despite these and other efforts by local councils to have extra resources allocated to them for community based services, the amendment made merely authorized a change in the wording of the Welfare Services Act (NI) 1949, so that people suffering from a mental disorder would be included among recipients of residential accommodation and domestic help. (Sect. 81)

The second lobby, which was much more highly orchestrated than the community care lobby, was for the establishment of a special unit for mentally ill offenders. In its final form, the Act gave permissive power to the Hospitals Authority to provide special accommodation for violent or dangerous patients. (Sect. 80) This was to satisfy the demands of the Northern Ireland Association for Mental Health, the BMA (NI Branch), and the Mental Health Services Committee of the Hospitals Authority. (NIHC Deb. 1961, Col. 2650) The arguments being put forward by these bodies were similar. Patients requiring a high level of security were an impediment to the 'open door' policies being encouraged in mental hospitals. According to Bessie Maconaghie, a barrister representing Queen's University :

If we are accepting a situation that the mental hospital is gradually becoming integrated with the whole hospital service, we have got to accept the further point of view that there are persons who will have to be looked after in a particular way. They present serious problems for the hospitals. (NIHC Deb. 1961, Col. 2647)

The Ministry was unwilling to build a special unit for offender patients because of the small numbers involved. During the only period when there had been a specially designated criminal lunatic asylum for

Northern Ireland at Derry Prison (from 1930 to 1945) the number had never exceeded eight. Understandably, the Ministry was reluctant to embark on a project involving unecessary expense. However, the lobby was not entirely unsuccessful as the Act allowed for possible developments. When the Act received Royal Assent on 19 December 1961, it was acceptable to most of the people who had been involved in the consultation process. If there was any dissatisfaction, it concerned the lack of a clear mandate for the development of community care services.

Implementation

The main elements of the Mental Health Act (NI) 1961 were: 1) The introduction of 'formal' (compulsory) and 'informal' (voluntary) admission procedures and the complete abolition of certification (by a judicial authority). (Part 2) ; 2) The establishment of a Mental Health Review Tribunal for Northern Ireland. (Part 6); 3) Permissive powers given to the Hospitals Authority to open a special unit for 'dangerous, violent or criminal' patients. (Part 7); and 4) Permissive powers given to the Hospitals Authority to fund organizations engaged in the promotion of mental health. (Part 1)

The new Act, like its counterparts in England (1959) and Scotland (1960), incorporated most of the recommendations of the Percy Commission (HMSO 1957) including a further informalization of admission to hospital care; the provision of new mechanisms for protecting the rights of detained patients; and an acknowledgment of the special problem of the care of offenders with mental disorders. Underlying these trends was an acceptance of an enlargement of the role of the medical profession in dealing with mental disorder and a lessening of the role of the legal profession.

Because the Act was a development of the earlier one, its implementation was relatively problem free. Procedures for admission to hospital were simpler than those in the English Act. Voluntary admissions posed no problem as they were similar to general hospital admissions. For patients who refused treatment there was a formal admission procedure for an initial 21 days, with the possibility of extending it for an additional six months, and an emergency admission procedure for seven days. (Sect. 12 & 15) Application for both types of admission could be made by the nearest relative or by a 'duly authorized' welfare officer supported by one medical certificate. In the case of an emergency admission the welfare officer could make the application without the permission of the nearest relative (which was required for the ordinary formal admission). The English Act stipulated three types of compulsory admission – for observation, for treatment and in an emergency situation. (Mental Health

Act 1959, Sect. 25-29) In the case of the first two, application for admission could be made by a Mental Welfare Officer or by the nearest relative, supported by two medical certificates. The emergency order required only one medical certificate. The immediate effect of the Act was to increase the proportion of voluntary (now called informal) admissions to hospital. The following chart shows the pattern of admissions before and after 1961.

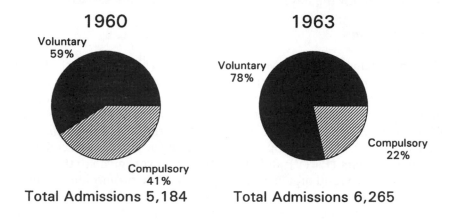

Figure 4.4   Legal status of admissions to mental hospitals 1960 and 1963

Source: HMSO (NI) 1961; HMSO (NI) 1964

This trend continued during the following years with an overall decrease in compulsory (now called formal) patients in hospital. Other aspects of the legislation developed at a more uneven pace. The new Mental Health Tribunal, chaired by F.A.L. Harrison Q.C., which was responsible for monitoring compulsory admissions, received more appeals in its first year of operation than it did in the second. The numbers were small however, when one considers the numbers of potential applicants for those years. In 1962, a total of 42 patients appealed to the Tribunal and in 1963 only 28 ventured to do so. This constituted four per cent of formal admissions in the first year and two per cent in the second year. It would take some time before people realized the potential value of the Tribunal. The special unit for dangerous and criminal mental patients permitted under the new legislation never materialized. During the years immediately following the passing of the 1961 Act, there were numerous consultations between the Ministry of Health and Local Government, the Hospitals Authority and Trade Unions, in an effort to resolve the problem of managing these patients in the ordinary hospital setting. [HMSO(NI) 1964, p. 15; NIHA 1954, p. 18] Because of the small numbers involved and against the wishes of the Unions, the Ministry decided not to approve the opening of a special unit. Instead, arrangements were made to transfer very difficult patients to Carstairs Hospital in Scotland.

The development of community based services was extremely slow. The Act had not given any clear mandate to local authorities to develop either preventive or rehabilitative services. However, section 2(a) did give the Hospitals Authority power to 'contribute towards the expenses of any organization having for its objects, or among its principle objects, the promotion of mental health or the welfare of persons suffering from mental disorder'. This positive statement was welcomed by the Northern Ireland Association for Mental Health (NIAMH), the only voluntary organization in this sphere. The Association had already received initial funding from the Ministry of Health and Local Government (NIAMH Minutes 16/12/59) and plans were underway for the opening of an advice centre and of a hostel. The centre, Beacon House, opened in Belfast in 1962, with affiliated clubs opening in other parts of the Province later on in the decade. It aimed to help patients make adjustments between hospital and home by offering support and advice in dealing with practical as well as emotional problems. (NIAMH Minutes 8/10/62) Funding by the Hospitals Authority ensured the continuity of Beacon House and other projects aimed at developing public interest and support in the promotion of mental health.

The NIAMH was important not only because of the projects it developed for discharged patients, but because it also played a major educational role in relation to mental health during the early 1960s. The first executive committee represented influential legal, medical and political opinion within the Province. Lady Wakehurst (wife of the Governor for Northern Ireland) was the founder and active President of the Association. Other influential people included Mr Justice Mc Veigh (Chairman 1959-65), Bessie Maconaghie, MP for Queen's University and also a member of the legal profession and John G. Gibson, Professor of Mental Health. As well as organizing public meetings, the Association was involved frequently in discussions with the Ministry. (NIAMH Minutes 1959-63)

The message given to local authorities by the new legislation was less positive. The decision to use an amendment to the Welfare Services Act (NI) 1949 as a means of ensuring local authority involvement in services for mentally ill people, was seen by many as a lack of commitment to the expansion of such services. The welfare committees of county and county borough councils could ignore this section of the Act without any fear of reprisal. In contrast to the legislation in Northern Ireland, the English

Mental Health Act 1959 made explicit the principles outlined in the National Health Service Act 1946 by authorizing local authorities to provide residential and day care facilities, in addition to 'ancilliary or supplementary services for the benefit of persons who are or have been suffering from mental disorder'. [Sect. 28(1)] Local councils in England and Wales were encouraged to play a significant role in the development of community based services while in Northern Ireland the highly centralized Hospitals Authority continued to be the major provider of mental health services.

Efforts by the Ministry to initiate local projects failed. In 1959 in a letter to local health authorities the Ministry urged the use of health visitors in the mental health services. (NIHA 1960, p. 64) In June of the following year it again issued a circular on *Local Authority Services for the Sick and Handicapped* explaining that :

> ... the development of local authority mental health services could not be dissociated from the development of other health and welfare services by local authorities, and such authorities were, therefore, asked to consider ways in which mental health services and services for ill or handicapped persons in general could be developed in the community. (NIHA 1960, p. 64)

However, welfare committees during the 1950s were concerned primarily with the provision of residential accommodation for children and old people displaced by the closure of workhouses. Having successfully transferred responsibily for mental hospitals to central government in 1948, local councils were unwilling to accept any responsibility for mental health services. This was shown clearly in relation to elderly patients in mental hospitals. Wrangling between hospital management committees and county welfare committees usually ended by the former being reminded that the responsibility was their's under Section 74 of the Mental Health Act (NI) 1948. [PRO(NI) HSS 16/6/156] This area of provision, which could have been the focus of cooperation between the Hospitals Authority and local councils did not develop. Though reports of the Hospitals Authority in the late 1950s referred to cooperation with local authorities, this was mainly in relation to the Special Care Service. It was not until the late 1960s that any concerted effort was made by councils to plan hostels and day centres for patients with mental illnesses.

In summary, the impact of the Mental Health Act (NI) 1961 was one of incremental rather than radical change. It was the last link in the chain of health service developments which had begun with the Health Services Act (NI) 1948. The new legislation, in simplifying legal procedures, made services more accessible and was received with great enthusiasm by mental health professionals, who saw it as the final nail in the coffin of nineteenth century treatment of mental disorder.

Discussion

This was a period during which the political promises of the post-war era came true. Northern Ireland experienced almost two decades of relative peace and stability and in spite of the decline of the major industries and the continuing high levels of unemployment, the standard of living rose as public expenditure boosted education, housing and health services. The Northern Ireland government had the time and the financial resources to devote to social and economic development. For the mental health services, this was a time of major expansion. This expansion had some negative features, but these were not always immediately apparent. The expansion in bed numbers was in response to increasing numbers of people using the services during the 1950s. This increase was taken as a signal that mental disorder was losing its stigma. The possible negative effects of segregation and institutionalization of large groups of people were not yet debated.

The major moving force in hospital developments during this time, the Northern Ireland Hospitals Authority, introduced rational if bureaucratic planning and decision making into the Northern Ireland health services. Not since the heyday of the Inspectorate of Lunacy at Dublin Castle during the 1860s had the mental hospitals experienced such tight controls over decision making. Management committees were naive enough to think that they could have the best of both worlds – a high degree of central funding and a high degree of local autonomy. After an initial period of difficult communication, the balance between central and local control seems to have been achieved and hospitals were free to develop new services within the framework of general guidelines. The dominance of the Hospitals Authority in health service provision continued throughout the period, in spite of efforts by the Ministry to promote community care initiatives. The lack of development of mental health services by local authorities had repercussions for many years. The concept of caring for or treating mental illness from a community base had not yet gained general social approval.

As the 1960s progressed, some of the problems which were to dominate the next decade began to appear. Some were similar to those in other areas of the United Kingdom and some were different. Northern Ireland, because of its geographical isolation from England and its political isolation from the rest of Ireland, could not rely on either England or the Republic of Ireland for a supply of qualified health care staff. Though the numbers would be small the only solution seemed to be the development of training courses within the Province for all the health professions. This was both expensive and difficult. The second problem was the high cost of modern hospital treatment. Because of the lack of information on health services prior to 1948 and because of the state of underdevelopment of these services, projected costs had been grossly underestimated. As the possibility of community based treatment for mental illness became a reality, the question of comparative costs became important. Initiatives such as the day hospital and hostel accommodation were viewed very positively as cheaper alternatives to hospital treatment.

The final issue to emerge was that of the loss of local control as a consequence of the acceptance of central funding. This applied on two levels. The Northern Ireland government, by reaping the benefits of 'welfare state' policies from the United Kingdom lost autonomy in relation to policy decisions on public expenditure. At local level councils had lost responsibility for mental hospitals in 1948 and the elected hospital management committees found that they had little control in the context of the powerful Hospitals Authority. However, though there were problems there was also satisfaction that steady progress was being made in the development of a modern mental health service. As the 1960s progressed, the right of Northern Ireland citizens to the same benefits and services as existed in other parts of the United Kingdom was taken for granted. But as education, health and housing improved, some sections of the community realized that the right of a citizen to services did not necessarily imply equality of access to them.

5 The 'troubles' and mental health

> Eleven people were killed and 63 injured, 19 of them seriously, when a bomb planted yards from the cenotaph in Enniskillen, County Fermanagh, turned the small country town's Remembrance Day into a scene of carnage . . . No organization claimed responsibility yesterday, but the Chief Constable, Sir John Hermon, said he was in no doubt that the IRA was responsible. (The Guardian, 9 November 1987)

Since 1969 the people of Northern Ireland have been exposed to incidents such as this one. Some of the people of Enniskillen will never recover from this bombing. Their lives have been shattered by the death or serious injury of a friend or relative. Others, because at that precise moment they happened to be in a different part of the town are alive and well. Like other atrocities, this aroused feelings of grief, anger and a desire for revenge among the people of Enniskillen and of towns and villages all over the Province. This time the IRA were responsible.

Other violent incidents came from the opposite side of the political divide. The following newspaper report tells of one of the major incidents in the cluster of spiralling violence during March 1988.

> An extreme loyalist paramilitary group, the Protestant Action Force, last night claimed responsibility for the killing of the three mourners shot yesterday at the funeral in Milltown cemetery, Belfast, of the three IRA bombers shot by the SAS in Gibralter 10 days ago . . . . The RUC was last night questioning two men following the grenade and gun attack, in which 68 people were injured, two of them seriously . . . . The gunman walked from the nearby motorway towards the republican plot in the cemetery and lobbed five grenades into the 20,000 strong crowd just as the third of the coffins was being lowered into the joint plot. (The Guardian 17 March 1988)

The thousands of people who attended this funeral were involved in this incident. As the grenades came hurtling towards the crowd many were not only terrified by the attack itself but by the possibility of being crushed to death in the panic. One wonders what will be the psychological effects of this experience on these people. Will they have nightmares or develop phobias? After the initial panic was over did they go to their doctor for tranquillizers, or will they feature in mental health statistics sometime in the future?

These are some of the questions which have been asked constantly since the beginning of the 'troubles' in Northern Ireland over twenty years ago. The purpose of the following discussion is to examine the relationship between the civil disturbances at the height of the 'troubles' and developments in the mental health policy, to assess the impact of one on the other. There are two distinct questions to be answered before any conclusions can be drawn. How did the serious rioting and political upheaval of the late 1960s and early 1970s affect the mental health of the population and did the violence have any effect on the planning or delivery of mental health services during or after this period?

Political violence

Under British rule Northern Ireland has never been free from political unrest. The presence of two communities, each with its own cultural identity and value system, provides a constant basis for potential conflict. There were sporadic outbreaks of violence in the 1920s (with 361 deaths in 1922), in the 1930s (15 deaths in 1935) and in the mid 1950s (12 deaths between 1956 and 1962). (Thompson 1989, p. 680) However, it was not until the late 1960s that continuous street violence became a part of the daily reality of many people, especially those living in the cities of Belfast and Derry.

The roots of the dissension may lie in the plantation of Ulster by Scottish Presbyterians but the current situation arises out of the geographic proximity of two communities with opposing ideologies. The origins of the last phase of violence can be traced to the establishment in 1967, of the Northern Ireland Civil Rights Association (NICRA). This association, born of the frustration felt by the Catholic minority, had among its aims the procurement of fairer local council elections, the establishment of machinery to prevent discrimination by public authorities, and the abolition of what was seen as an unfair method of housing allocation. (Buckland 1981, p. 118) NICRA, influenced by the civil rights movement in America and modelled on the London based National Council for Civil Liberties, did not see itself as a nationalist organization.

[HMSO(NI) 1969b, para. 12] However, this was a difficult boundary to draw as the majority of its members were Catholic. The first civil rights march in August 1968 passed off peacefully. The second, on the 5th October of the same year, was the scene of intense violent clashes between police and marchers. Seventy eight civilians and eighteen policemen were injured. (Buckland 1981, p. 122) Thus began a period of civil disturbance which took both the population at large and those in authority by surprise.

Political attempts to change the situation did not stem the violence which followed the NICRA march. In May 1969 James Chichester Clark replaced Terence O'Neill as Prime Minister for Northern Ireland. In the same month Stormont issued a White Paper on the *Reshaping of Local Government.* [HMSO(NI) 1969a] The existing 73 local councils, accused by NICRA of blatant discrimination against the Catholic minority in the allocation of housing and jobs, were to be replaced by 17 new councils with no responsibility for education, health or welfare services. These services would be administered in future by area boards. (Ibid. paras. 16-17) This meant that powers taken from elected local councils were given to appointed professionals. The promise of reform did not stop the serious rioting which occurred in August – just one month after the publication of the White Paper. The British government was to learn in the years which followed, that social reform alone would never lead to peace in Northern Ireland, but in 1969 this was not so clear.

The escalation of the violence was not due to social and economic deprivation alone but to the political context of the time. (For discussion see Thompson 1989, p. 686) The rioting which took place in August 1969 was precipitated not only by the allegations of discrimination made by NICRA but also by the 'marching season' traditional to Northern Ireland. The annual march of the Apprentice Boys (one of the Protestant 'loyal Orders') in Derry on 12 August was attacked by a group of Catholic youths. These youths were followed into the Catholic Bogside area by the Royal Ulster Constabulary (RUC), thus sparking off a riot which spread quickly throughout the city. Rioting followed in the towns of Dungannon, Dungiven, Lurgan, Newry and Armagh. Serious rioting also took place in Belfast, with units of the British Army intervening between the Falls Road and the Shankill Road, establishing what later became known as the 'Peace Line'. [Darby & Williamson (eds) 1978, p. xii]

Before the end of that month, August 1969, the 'Downing Street Declaration' was issued jointly by the United Kingdom and Northern Ireland Governments outlining the principles for future action to ensure economic development. (HMSO 1969; Wilson 1989, p. 163))

During August also, the Home Secretary, James Callaghan, paid a three-day visit to the Province – appealing for calm and promising equality of citizenship to the Northern Ireland population. Two enquiries followed almost immediately – the Hunt Committee on the police and the Scarman Enquiry into the disturbances which had taken place in the Summer of 1969. [Harkness 1983, p. 160; HMSO(NI) 1969c; HMSO(NI) 1972]

A third enquiry was already underway – the Cameron Commission, appointed in March to examine the causes and nature of the civil disturbances since 5 October 1968, presented its report in September 1969. [HMSO(NI) 1969b] It acknowledged the existence of genuine grievances on the part of the minority community and recommended the 'honest implementation of reforms already promised or foreshadowed by the Government with the least necessary delay . . .' (Ibid. para. 232) In its reply the Northern Ireland Government affirmed its commitment to the sentiments expressed in the Cameron Report and outlined progress which had been made in the areas where discrimination had been alleged. [HMSO(NI) 1969b] In October the Hunt Report (on the police in Northern Ireland) made forty seven recommendations two of which were that the Royal Ulster Constabulary (RUC) be disarmed and that security should become a military responsibility. [HMSO(NI) 1969c, para. 183]

Following on the Cameron Report and the Hunt Report, a number of reforms were initiated immediately. A Community Relations Commission and a Commission for Complaints (Ombudsman's Office) were established in November 1969 and new legislation imposing penalties for incitement to riot was passed in July 1970. [The Prevention of Incitement to Hatred Act (NI)] In spite of these initiatives, street violence continued to escalate. James Chichester-Clarke resigned as Prime Minister in March 1971 and was replaced by Brian Faulkner.

> Faulkner set out . . . to bring the reform programme to fruition, to involve the new generation of minority representatives in the decision-making process, and to encourage his own uneasy back-benchers by the resolute defeat of unlawful activity. (Harkness 1983, p. 167)

However, constitutional change failed to stop the violence as can be seen from Figures 5.1 and 5.2. (See also Buckland 1981, p. 140) The consequent pressure on the government to take some action to restore peace led to the introduction of internment without trial on 9 August 1971. In a swoop named Operation Motorman, the Army picked up 645 people, interrogated them by methods subsequently repudiated by the British Government, and interned them on hulks in Belfast Lough. (Jones 1992)

This decision led to the sharp polarization of the two communities in Northern Ireland though there was an immediate decrease in terrorist activity. The population had scarcely recovered from the shock of Operation Motorman when the security forces, who were supposed to be preserving law and order, were again seen to flaunt the law in the name of order. The shooting of 13 young men in the Catholic Bogside of Derry on 30 January 1972 (a day which became known as 'Bloody Sunday') was seen as the final outrage by the Catholic community and as media images of paratroopers shooting indiscriminately at an unarmed crowd were flashed around the world, the British government came under intense pressure to intervene.

The Heath Government, determined to bring about change with or without the consent of the Northern Ireland Government, proposed the withdrawal of responsibility for security from Stormont. The Northern Ireland government found the Westminster proposal unacceptable and (on 24 March 1972) it resigned rather than co-operate. Heath accepted the resignation and in the midst of controversy, Westminster assumed direct responsibility for the Province. The Northern Ireland (Temporary Provisions) Act 1972 suspended the Stormont Parliament, initially for one year, and appointed William Whitelaw as the Secretary of State. Direct Rule had begun.

The situation reached crisis point as the number of individuals being caught up in the violence increased rapidly. (See Figures 5.1 and 5.2) The change in government strategy, signalled by the appointment of William Whitelaw as Secretary of State, did not stop the violence. Indeed bombings and killings escalated during 1972. The year will be remembered for being the worst year of violence, with the number of deaths reaching 467 (of whom 332 were civilians) and the number of injuries 4,876. [HMSO(NI) 1973; Harkness 1983, p. 173] In an attempt to restore political stability, a new formula for governing was worked out and in January 1974 the Northern Ireland Executive, led by Brian Faulkner, took office. This genuine attempt at power sharing, involving six Unionists, four member of the Social Democratic Liberal Party (SDLP), and one Alliance party member, proved powerless in the face of opposition from the Ulster Workers Council which called a general strike in May. After less than five months in power the Executive resigned, and Direct Rule from Westminster was restored. [Harkness 1983, p. 173; Darby and Williamson (eds) 1978, p. xv]

During the years immediately following the imposition of Direct Rule, the violence continued but never again reached the 1972 peak. The following charts show deaths and injuries during this period and afterwards.

101

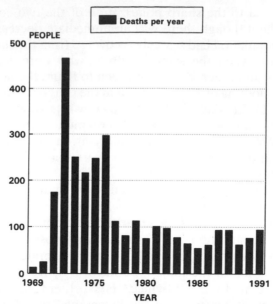

Figure 5.1 Deaths due to political violence in Northern Ireland 1969-91

Source: Annual abstract of statistics

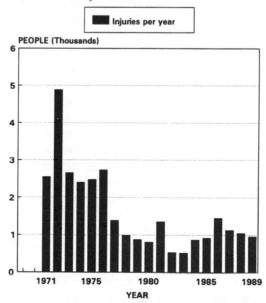

Figure 5.2 Injuries due to political violence in Northern Ireland 1971-89

Source: Annual abstract of statistics

While the saga of death and destruction continued, the new leadership made attempts to speed up the reforms already promised. In 1973 a Standing Advisory Committee on Human Rights was established, as was a working party on Discrimination in the Private Sector of Employment under the direction of William Van Straubenzee (Minister of State for Northern Ireland). On the recommendation of the Van Straubenzee Report, a Fair Employment Agency was established in 1974. (Wilson 1989, p. 119) In December 1975, on the recommendation of the Gardiner Committee (HMSO 1975b), internment without trial was finally abolished and the last of the detainees were released from the Maze Prison. In spite of these developments the violence continued, with an increase in the numbers of dead and injured during the following year. However, the situation continued to ease somewhat as the 1970s drew to a close and reached what some people viewed as an 'acceptable level of violence'. Understandably, for those bereaved or injured by the violence there can never be an 'acceptable level'. Their lives have been disrupted in a way which can never be forgotten.

Political violence and mental health

Opinions on the impact of the 'troubles' on the people of Northern Ireland are divided. Newspaper reports during the early stages of the intensive rioting indicated a massive onslaught on the psychiatric services. The following is a typical example of these reports.

> A serious wave of mental illness has developed in Belfast as a result of last week's rioting and continued tension. Doctors are reporting influxes of patients with mental breakdowns. In some cases, the symptoms are so severe that they have had to be admitted to mental hospitals . . . one doctor in the Shankill Road area – the scene of one of Belfast's most bitter fights – said he had prescribed more tranquillizing drugs in the past five days than he usually does in a year . . . . A spokeman for Purdysburn Mental Hospital estimated that since the riots, admissions had increased by 25 per cent. People who had been burned out of their houses and who had been taken into the city's makeshift refugee centres had, in some cases, completely broken down. They were chiefly suffering from anxiety states and reactive depression. In two cases men had been admitted who had become obsessed by the fear that they were going to be shot . . .
> (The Guardian, 23 August 1971)

A number of other newspaper reports in September 1971 carried statements from GPs on the increase in people suffering from tension and seeking tranquillizers. (See Fraser 1974, p. 65) The academic literature reveals a slightly different and more complex picture. The psychological effects of street violence and political unrest have been the subject of a number of studies by psychiatrists and psychologists in Northern Ireland. In a review article on the psychiatric aspects of terrorist violence, Dr Peter Curran, psychiatrist at the Mater Hospital in Belfast, outlines the methodological difficulties involved in measuring these effects. (Curran 1988) They include the definition of the population to be studied; the choice of measuring instruments; the decision about the timing of the research and finally, the choice of expert. In spite of these difficulties, studies have been carried out at different times using varied methods of measurement and different target populations. Studies by Dr R. M. Fraser (1971 and 1974), a child psychiatrist working for the Northern Ireland Hospitals Authority, and Dr H. A. Lyons (1971), a psychiatrist at Purdysburn Hospital, Belfast, documented the immediate effects of the violence in 1969. Fraser (1974) in the first major study to examine the 'psychiatric sequelae' of the violence found that there was evidence of two types of psychiatric ill health. The first, the 'acute emotional reactions seen in people who had been directly exposed to riot conditions', normally resolved when the 'troubles' ceased or when the person had received mild sedation. (p. 81) The second, psychiatric illness requiring admission to hospital, showed a significant increase 'only in areas adjacent to those affected by rioting'. (Fraser 1971, p. 263 and 1974, p. 81)

Lyons (1971), in a study carried out during the most intensive period of rioting, from August 15 to the end of September 1969, found no increase in acute psychotic illness. Those who developed symptoms 'tended either to develop a short lived 'normal anxiety' reaction or, in those with a previous psychiatric history, the illness pattern usually repeated itself'. (Lyons 1971, p. 272) Lyons' results were based on interviews with 217 patients from three GP practices in West Belfast (centre of the riot area). Each of these patients had attended or had requested a psychiatric appointment during the period of study. In his second study one year later, Lyons examined the incidence of depressive illness in Belfast and suicide rates for the whole of Northern Ireland. He found a significant decrease in the incidence of depressive illness during the 1969-70 period when compared with the 1964-68 period. (Lyons 1972, p. 343) He also found that the suicide rate had dropped dramatically in 1970-72, at the same time as the homicide rate increased. He inferred from these findings that the increased opportunities afforded by the situation allowed people to externalize aggressive impulses and that this reduced the incidence of depressive illness and suicide. In contrast to these findings, Dr P. O'Malley (1969), psychiatrist at the Mater Hospital in West Belfast, found a significant increase in admissions of attempted suicides to the hospital.

These early studies have been examined in the light of later research in Northern Ireland, and of international literature on the effects of civil disorder, riots and terrorism. (Loughrey and Curran 1987; Trew 1987; Cairns and Wilson 1989)

The international literature generally provides evidence against an increase in psychiatric morbidity or admissions during civil disorder or war although the evidence regarding outpatient referrals is contradictory, some sources implying a rebound increase later. (Loughrey and Curran 1987, p. 4)

On the suicide statistics the general view is that one cannot draw any conclusions from the findings of either Lyons (1972) or O' Malley (1969) as suicide rates in England and Wales also dropped during the early 1970s (Cairns and Wilson 1989, p. 44); suicide statistics are notoriously unreliable among Catholic populations; and there is little likelihood of a correlation between suicide and homicide as people who commit suicide do not generally turn to homicide or vice versa. (Loughrey and Curran 1987, p. 6)

Later studies used more rigorous methodologies and also focused on broader themes. King et al (1977 and 1982) carried out two studies on the prescription rates for psychotropic drugs. The second study, which was based on the computerized pricing data for prescriptions in Northern Ireland from 1966 to 1980 'showed that the use of these drugs reached a peak in 1975, when about 12.5 per cent of the adult population were estimated to have been receiving them, and declined in the following five years'. (King et al. 1982, p. 819) When compared with similar figures for other Western European countries, the Northern Ireland prescription rates were not notably higher. The authors found no evidence of a direct relationship between tranquillizer prescribing in the Province as a whole and the severe rioting from 1969 to 1972 although they did acknowledge that the possibility of long term effects of those civil disturbances could not be ruled out. It was more likely, they argued, that the overall trends in psychotropic drug use were following world wide changes in prescribing patterns and patient demand. The effect of civil disturbances was not tested directly but one of the variables used in the study was an index of population movement. Because of the existing literature on migration as a factor in the aetiology of mental illness and because of the extensive population movements caused by the street violence in the 1969-74 period, the authors were surprised to find no relationship between population movements and psychotropic prescription levels.

In a recent retrospective survey of a large number of people who each had been a victim of terrorist violence, Loughrey and Curran found that

... 66 per cent had been prescribed tranquillizers, 42 per cent hypnotics and 13 per cent anti-depressants and that approximately one third of the total sample had taken psychotropic drugs for longer than 12 months. (Loughrey and Curran 1987, p. 10)

This finding, which seems to contradict that of King et al. (1982), is in keeping with international evidence (and indeed with early newspaper reports) that there is some evidence of an increase in the consumption of tranquillizers in urban areas during times of civil unrest. It is very difficult to assess these findings because not only have the patterns of prescribing and of violence changed since the early 1970s, but so also have social attitudes to tranquillizers. Republican prisoners in the Maze prison told members of the Gardiner Committee of their fear of tranquillizers for themselves and for their womenfolk. They were particularly afraid of the possibility of Librium in the water (of the prison) in case it would destroy their will to carry on the struggle and women from Catholic areas who took tranquillizers were under threat of being tarred and feathered. (Jones 1992) As women are thought to be more vulnerable to stress than men in these situations (King et al. 1982, p. 830; Loughrey and Curran 1987, p. 9) then this attitude could have artificially suppressed the demand for tranquillizers during the early 1970s.

A further study, carried out in 1983 by two psychologists, Cairns and Wilson (1984), focused on a different theme. They decided to concentrate on 'mild psychiatric morbidity' and to do this using community-based samples. (Cairns & Wilson 1984, p. 632) The two areas chosen were representative of parts of Northern Ireland which had experienced differing levels of recorded violence. Hitown had experience a high level of violence and Lotown a low level. Respondents (797) from the two chosen towns were interviewed in July and August 1983, using the General Health Questionnaire (GHQ) and questions aimed at showing their perception of the level of violence in their area. The results indicated that 'the majority of people in Northern Ireland manage to deal effectively with stress generated by the troubles, but that a small minority are at risk'. Those most at risk were those who were conscious of the violence. The authors conclude that 'denial of reality is for the people of certain areas of Northern Ireland at least one way to remain stable in a threatening environment'. (Ibid. p. 635)

Dr P. Curran, acknowledged expert in this field, suggests that in spite of some slightly contradictory findings, the evidence in all of the psychiatric literature points to the fact that the street violence and political unrest have not 'resulted in any obvious increase in psychiatric morbidity.' (Curran 1988, p. 473) He offers some possible reasons for this rather surprising finding. Perhaps people don't report their symptoms or feelings because they feel nothing can be done for them; migration from the troubled areas may have been selective of the psychologically vulnerable; people may use denial as a defense against an intolerable reality; participation in the violence may have a cathartic effect; people with neurotic symptoms may have improved when faced with external stress, and finally the sense of common purpose and common outrage may have bonded people together. (Ibid. pp. 473-75)

One of these explanations at least has been shown to have validity in the Northern Ireland situation – people use denial as their only means of psychological survival in situations which are intolerable and over which they have no control. (Cairns and Wilson 1984) This can be done by avoiding media coverage of violence, by not going into 'troubled' areas and by refusing to take part in discussions on anything remotely connected to the violence. Adaptation to stress by using different coping mechanisms such as denial is characteristic of all animals (including humans). (Heskin 1980, p. 67) What is not known is the extent of the cumulative psychological cost of this adaptation.

Another suggested reason for the apparent improvement in the mental health of at least some of the population during political violence is that frank mental illness gets cloaked by military and para military activity. Heskin (1980, p. 78) examines the assertion 'that terrorist groups contain strong psychopathic elements' in relation to the IRA, and argues against it. However, he points out that this in not to argue that there are no 'psychopathic' individuals in these organizations.

> Psychopathic individuals may be attracted to conflict-oriented groups to indulge themselves with impunity, and indeed, in the short term, may be useful to such organizations . . . In the long term, however, their egocentricity and unreliability would make them a dangerous liability to such an organization . . . (Heskin 1980, p. 83)

The absorbtion of some aggressive behaviour into paramilitary activity cannot be denied but it cannot be advanced as a reason for the seemingly inverse relationship between political violence and mental health admissions and referrals.

As more recent studies (on the psychological effects of violence immediately after it happens) have shown, there is another factor at work. (Kee et al. 1987; Loughrey et al. 1988; Curran et al. 1990) It is the extent to which emotional or psychological disturbance is looked for among people exposed to violence. Hadden et al. (1978, p. 529) in a study of 1,532 victims of terrorist bombings, found that 50 per cent of patients had psychological disturbances. The more recent studies, using internationally accepted methods of measuring post traumatic stress disorder (developed after the Vietnam War by the American Psychiatric Association) and measures from the General Health Questionnaire (GHQ), have focussed on people at different stages of recovery after bombings or shootings. (Curran et al. 1990, p. 479: Loughrey et al. 1988, p. 559) After the bombing in Enniskillen in November 1987, in which 11 people were killed and 60 injured, 37 survivors were assessed six months and one year later. At six months 50 per cent had developed post traumatic stress disorder (PTSD) and only one had recovered six months later. (Curran et al. 1990, p. 480) Whether or not these people will recover completely without psychiatric intervention is not clear. What is significant is the fact that they are being studied.

Many people of course never come to the attention of researchers and some are reluctant to take part in studies. Dillenburger (1992, p. 52) achieved only a 36 per cent return rate in her study of widows whose husbands had been killed in the 'troubles'. Her findings give us some valuable insights into the factors which affected the recovery of the 67 widows who took part in the study – three of the most important being the income level of the widow, the duration of the marriage before the husband's death and the 'the way in which the death message was communicated'. (Ibid. p. 67) Though the author used the General Health Questionnaire (GHQ) as her main measuring instrument (Ibid., pp. 49-50), she confuses the reader by interchanging terms such as 'psychiatric distress', 'psychiatric health', 'psychological distress' and 'psychological health' in her discussion of the GHQ scores. However, it is clear from the study that the violent death of a spouse is a devastating experience even for those for whom it is a daily risk (security force personnel) and that an open acknowledgment of this grief is a step on the road to recovery. How many thousands of people in the towns and cities of Northern Ireland have been exposed to gunfire, bombs and riots without any help in coping with the stress except for that provided by family? The need for disaster planning to ensure the provision of crisis intervention services during a violent incident and counselling services afterwards is now acknowledged. (See Gibson 1991) In the 1970s, however, this was not the case.

Policy developments

Ditch and Morrissey (1979, p. 214) were of the opinion that 'It is not possible for a guerilla war to be conducted for a decade within a welfare state without profound implications for social policy'. At first glance it looks as if they were wrong in relation to mental health policy. Annual reports of the Northern Ireland Hospitals Authority for the period 1968-73 (when the violence was at its height) referred to it only in connection with the ambulance services in Belfast and Derry, which were put under severe pressure during the riots in August and September 1969. (NIHA Report for 1969, p. 50) Neither did the major survey of psychiatric facilities, carried out by Dr S. N. Donaldson in 1975, take into account the political situation or the ongoing civil strife. This lack of acknowledgment of the existence of a crisis situation fits neatly with the general pattern of denial observed in the psychiatric literature. It also fits international patterns of demand (or the lack of it) for mental health services during riots or war. In contrast, other services such as welfare, housing and general hospital casualty departments, experienced serious disruptions and increased demand. (Herron and Caul 1992)

The number and frequency of casualties put the hospital services in Belfast under severe strain. The Royal Victoria Hospital, for example, made regular use of the disaster drill during the period of intensive bombing and street burning. Housing policy was affected at every level. Massive population movements within Belfast completely disrupted plans for ongoing housing developments.

> After three days of rioting in August 1969, 4,000 people left their homes and 500 houses were made uninhabitable. In the most serious single incident an entire street was burnt out. (Ditch and Morrissey 1979, p. 217)

Fear of intimidation led to a massive increase in the population of West Belfast which in turn prompted the building of a new housing estate (designated for Catholics) on the outskirts of Belfast. This kind of change in house building plans had repercussions on all other housing projects in the Province. The personal social services, which until 1973 were the responsibility of Welfare Departments of local councils, were also put under severe strain. According to Herron and Caul (1992), the events appeared as a series of waves of violence with lulls in between. The 'troubles' were not a single entity, rather 'the tactics which terrorists adopted were constantly changing and these changes created new problems for social workers'. (Ibid. p. 103) For example, the first wave of rioting in August 1969 left many people homeless or injured or both. Access to many streets was difficult because of barricades and debris. A different set of problems emerged at Easter 1970, during the evacuation of a Protestant housing estate in West Belfast. Fear of a sectarian confrontation led to panic which sent women and children scurrying to the safety of schools. Social workers were involved in all of these events giving practical and emotional support. (Ibid. pp. 102-7)

The same immediacy of demand was not present in relation to mental health services. Staff of psychiatric hospitals and units were protected from the immediate impact of the crises to which their colleagues in housing and social services were exposed. They had to wait to see what would be the long term effects of the 'troubles'. The discussion cannot end here, however, as the imposition of Direct Rule and the major re-organization of local authority services during the early 1970s affected mental health policy directly. Plans for administrative reform within the public services were already underway before the outbreak of violence in 1969, but the immediate impact of the violence on these plans was to radicalize and expedite them.

Housing was the first major public service to be transferred from local councils to a new formed centralized authority (the Northern Ireland Housing Executive). This took place in 1970. Three years later all health and welfare responsibilities were re-allocated to Area Health and Social Services Boards. At the same time local authorities also lost responsibility for education and public libraries to new Area Education and Library Boards. Because of the significance of the re-organization of the health and social services for mental health policy during the following two decades, it is important to look at it in some detail.

A new structure for health and welfare

The re-organization of the health and personal social services in Northern Ireland arose out of two debates which took place during the 1960s. One centred around the demand within Northern Ireland for the re-organization of local government services and the other around the need for radical change in the structure of the NHS within the United Kingdom. The need for reform of the local government system in Northern Ireland had emerged initially in 1963 in the report of the Matthew Committee – a committee appointed to carry out an economic survey and draw up a regional plan for the Belfast area. [HMSO(NI) 1963] According to this report, the existing local government structure lacked the potential for the encouragement of regional and economic development. In 1967 the White Paper on the *Reshaping of Local Government* confirmed the commitment of Stormont to 'effective representation of local aspirations' as well as to economy and efficiency. [HMSO(NI) 1967] Further proposals on reform followed in July 1969. [HMSO(NI) 1969a] As the first Green Paper on the *Administrative Structure of the Health Services* had just been published in Britain (HMSO 1968a), it was also proposed that discussions should begin on a new structure for an integrated health service in Northern Ireland.

In August 1969, the month which witnessed the most extreme outbreak of political violence, a Green Paper on the *Administration of the Health and Personal Social Services in Northern Ireland* was published. [HMSO(NI) 1969d] The Green Paper acknowledged that the impetus for change within health services structures came from England as did

110

also the recommendation for the establishment of comprehensive social services departments. (HMSO 1968b) However, because of the potential impact of local government re-organization on existing health and welfare structures in Northern Ireland, the Ministry could not wait for the outcome of pilot projects in England. It was suggested at first that modification of the existing system might be sufficient, but this solution was rejected. 'Nothing short of a fully integrated administrative system can provide an adequate framework for comprehensive care today and for an effective response to the problems and challenges of tomorrow.' [HMSO(NI) 1969d, para. 24] Having accepted the principle of an integrated structure for health, a proposal for one or more Area Health Boards was outlined. To complement the health structure four models for social services were suggested, including one which allowed for continuing local authority control of social services. The model, with three to five Area Health and Social Services Boards, was regarded as the best option provided certain conditions were met. These were the establishment of two local committees, one for health and one for social services, the allocation of a budget and the appointment of a Chief Officer for Social Services. [Ibid. paras. 52-68]

Ihere was mixed reaction to these proposals. Local councils already knew of the public dissatisfaction with their administration of services. The Cameron Commission (appointed to inquire into civil disturbances in October 1968) had found that grievances in relation to the allocation of housing and the manipulation of electoral boundaries were justified.

> The weight and extent of the evidence which was presented to us, concerned with social and economic grievance or abuses of political power, was such that we are compelled to conclude that they had substantial foundation in fact and were in a real sense an immediate and operative cause of the demonstrations and consequent disorders after 5 October 1968. [HMSO(NI) 1969b, para. 127]

This report served only to confirm the failure of the Northern Ireland government to accept the reality of the discrimination being experienced by the Catholic minority and the urgent need for local government reform.

A joint communiqué, issued by Westminster and Stormont, on 10 October 1969 announced plans for the establishment of a central housing authority for Northern Ireland to initiate a new housing programme. (HMSO 1969) As housing was one of the most important functions held by local authorities, this announcement, in the words of the Macrory Review Body 'marked a radical departure from the existing system and introduced an entirely new factor into the re-shaping of local government'. [HMSO(NI) 1970, para. 19] The Macrory Review Body was appointed in December 1969 to review earlier proposals for the reform of local government, in the light of the decision on housing. In an effort to depoliticize local government services, Macrory proposed structures which would 'ensure professional standards' (Ibid. paras. 37-47) and suggested that education, health and social services would be best served by a system of Area Boards. This was the point of no return. Because of the ongoing political violence and because of the existence of evidence of misuse of local political power, local councils were in no position to argue for the retention of health or welfare services.

The debate on the need to retain local control over local services, a debate which has been clearly evident in the ongoing discussion in Britain on the need to re-organize the NHS, did not emerge in any public documentation in Northern Ireland during this period. The Seebohm Committee had rejected the idea of removing personal social services from local government.

> We see a high level of citizen participation as vital to the successful development of services which are sensitive to local needs, and we do not see how, at present, this participation can be achieved outside the local government system. (HMSO 1968b. para. 137)

In the Northern Ireland situation, citizen participation was taking such a violent form that the Government, unwilling to allow controversy and conflict in the areas of health and welfare, limited the role of elected representatives while involving professionals in the making of policy. In March 1971 the Ministry issued a consultative document on the *Restructuring of the Personal Health and Personal Social Services in Northern Ireland* [HMSO(NI) 1971] – the result of consultations which had taken place on the 1969 Green Paper [HMSO(NI) 1969d] in the context of local government reforms. The need for effective local involvement in the management of the services was acknowledged but it was also taken for granted that professional interests would be an intrinsic part of this structure.

> First we considered it essential that there should be effective local involvement, both through elected representation and otherwise, in the management of these very personal services. Second the new system had to recognize the established rights of certain interests to participate in management – for example . . . the medical profession in the administration of the health services. [HMSO(NI) 1971, para. 6]

Legislation passed in 1972 incorporated the main principles underlying this Consultative Document [Health and Personal Social Services (NI) Order 1972] and on the first of October 1973 the new system came into operation. Based on detailed plans drawn up by management consultants, Booz, Allen and Hamilton, four Health and Social Services Area Boards were established with responsibility for all health and welfare functions previously held by the Northern Ireland Hospitals Authority, the Northern Ireland General Health Services Board, the Special Care Service (NI) and by local authorities. (See Booz, Allen and Hamilton 1972) Three months later, as part of the devolution programme, under the Northern Ireland Constitution Act 1973, the Ministry for Health and Social Services (which had existed since 1965) was replaced by a Department of Health and Social Services which retained responsibility for health, personal social services and for social security.

The aim of this re-organization was not only to improve the quality of service to the consumer but to separate the delivery of health and social services from the political domain. The official view, within the DHSS(NI), was that the integration of health and social services was a progressive step.

> Northern Ireland has gone further than the rest of the United Kingdom, where responsibility for the provision of social services has remained the function of local government. The particular merit of the new structure is that it enables health and social services, especially for vulnerable groups such as the elderly, the mentally ill and the handicapped, to be planned and provided as a totality by one body within each area. [DHSS(NI) 1979, p. 6]

However, some aspects of the re-organization did not meet with unanimous approval. There were a number of difficulties with the new structures, difficulties which had long term negative effects on both the planning and delivery of services. Some of these difficulties were particularly apparent in the mental health services.

The first set of problems resulted from the replacement of a centralized hospitals authority with four Boards each with a broader mandate. Though the Hospitals Authority had been subjected to criticisms for its highly bureaucratic structure and its independence from proper political control, it had been responsible for extensive developments within hospitals. The psychiatric hospitals in the Province had derived particular benefit from the experience of being part of a centrally funded hospital service after a century of local government control. Since 1948 (when the Hospitals Authority was established), there had been improvements in hospital buildings, expansion of staffing levels (professional and non-professional), and significant improvements in services to patients. During the twenty five years of its existence the Hospitals Authority had streamlined its planning procedures and improved communications with individual hospital management committees. Furthermore, the Mental Health Services Committee (of the NIHA) had developed substantial expertize and knowledge in planning for mental health services. The replacement of these channels of communication and planning mechanisms took some time in the new Health and Social Services Boards.

The second set of problems came from the integration of health and social services. Mental health services consisted mainly of those initiated from the six psychiatric hospitals in the Province – inpatient and outpatient services from all hospitals, with developments of hostel accommodation and sheltered work schemes from some. The hostels were immediately separated administratively from the hospitals as they became the responsibility of the newly constituted Social Services Departments. As happened in England, staff from the social work departments in hospitals as well as welfare staff from local authority fieldwork offices merged to form these new departments.

In the upheaval which followed it often happened that the manager (Principal or Assistant Principal Social Worker) with responsibility for mental health hostels had little or no experience in mental health work, as the hostels were part of their overall responsibility for residential facilities for all client groups. Hostel managers (usually psychiatric nurses) who had been accustomed to close links with the hospital from which the patients had come, often found themselves being supervized by a social work manager whose knowledge of mental health was extremely limited. (Gregg 1990) Psychiatric social workers, who could have applied for these managerial positions often preferred not to do so, and remained in the protective atmosphere of the hospital. In Social Services offices outside the hospital setting, welfare officers with experience in mental health became part of a generic social work team with the consequent loss of this specialist knowledge. Statutory duties in relation to admissions and discharges under the existing mental health legislation, the Mental Health Act (NI) 1961, formed part of the role of senior social workers, the majority of whom had never worked in mental health.

In spite of these difficulties, the main outcome of the re-organization for the development of social services was positive. Social Services Departments expanded as more staff were employed and more facilities opened. This was due to increased public expenditure on health and social services following the introduction of Direct Rule in 1972. The re-organization of health and social services was only one aspect of the centralization of all the major social services in Northern Ireland between 1970 and 1973. This facilitated the imposition of more stringent control mechanisms from the Secretary of State through the expanded Northern Ireland Office (NIO) and Departmental structures. Public expenditure in Northern Ireland Departments had since 1968 been fitted into the United Kingdom Public Expenditure Survey Cycle (PESC), and the NIO expenditure became subject to its control procedure in 1972.

(O'Leary, Elliot and Wilford 1988, p. 64) As a separate Department of State (constituted as a result of Direct Rule in 1972) the NIO was successful in increasing public expenditure in the Province. From 1972 to 1979 Northern Ireland per capita public expenditure rose by 17 per cent compared with a rise of two per cent in Wales and an eight per cent reduction in Scotland. The impact of the extra money on mental health services was not immediately obvious but what was obvious was the different political environment within which the services would operate in the future.

Discussion

It is hard to imagine that any sphere of life in Northern Ireland would have been left unscathed by the political violence which began in 1969. However, an exploration of the psychiatric literature suggests that the demands made on the psychiatric services did not increase dramatically and that people seem to have coped well with intolerable situations. The main effect of the violence was to increase the pressure on the Stormont Government for reforms in the public service sector and in employment policies to ensure equal rights for all the citizens of Northern Ireland.

The imposition of Direct Rule from Westminster, on a temporary basis from March 1972 to December 1973, and on a permanent basis from May 1974, resulted in the speeding up of reforms in almost all areas of public service delivery. Among these reforms were the re-organization of health and social services under four Area Boards and the removal of any responsibility for these services from local councils. This re-organization and the interventionist style of government which has been in force in Northern Ireland since then has had a profound effect on mental health policy.

There are a number of questions which remain unanswered. Some of these have to do with the impact of the 'troubles' on the mental health of the people of Northern Ireland and others with the political changes which took place as a result of the 'troubles'. It is interesting that there has been no official acknowledgment of the need for special services for people who might be psychologically damaged by the political violence. How would the need for such a service be assessed? Perhaps some people are not legitimate targets for service planners. Who needs help after a bomb attack – the bystanders, the injured, the perpetrators or the security forces? How does need relate to demand? It may be that many victims of the Northern Ireland 'troubles' will never make any demand on services because of their commitment to the cause which has precipitated some of the violence. Can we expect demand to reflect need in

115

situations of such complexity? We can also ask – what will be the impact of the current situation on the mental health of the next generation – a situation in which people's rights are violated by searches and questioning, where negative attitudes to law and order and to state machinery prevail and where the population is exposed to ongoing violence.

It is difficult to speculate on what might have happened if the violence of the early 1970s had not occurred. Would local councils have retained control over welfare services, and if so how would this have affected the development of community based mental health services? And would public expenditure in Northern Ireland have increased at the same rate as it did under the new political structure? The answers to these questions will always be the subject of debate. What is certain is that the events of the turbulent years after 1969 radically changed the relationship between Britain and Northern Ireland. Control of political affairs within the Province was transferred from a locally elected Parliament to one elected by the people of the United Kingdom. Direct Rule from Westminster, introduced as a temporary measure, became the political norm, with successive Secretaries of State attempting to find solutions which would fit local needs while embodying the principles of British social policies.

6 Mental health policy under 'Direct Rule'

The impact of Direct Rule on social policy in Northern Ireland has been immense. Since 1972, with the exception of the period from 1982 to 1986 (when the Northern Ireland Assembly functioned) policy decisions have been made at Westminster and there has been no public forum for political debate on these decisions. One of the most striking differences in the style of government since 1972 is the fact that Ministers represent the orientation of the government in power in Westminster rather than the particular concerns of the Northern Ireland population. There have been nine Secretaries of State in Northern Ireland in that time, with a constantly changing group of junior Ministers. Civil servants, in a bureaucracy which has expanded to incorporate the new dimensions of governing from a distance, have handled the implementation of policies and local political debate on social and economic issues has virtually disappeared. The normal process of issue identification and policy formation has therefore been subverted in Northern Ireland and the probability of new issues or creative solutions emerging has almost disappeared. The context for policy making has moved firmly to Westminster in spite of the fact that the environment within which these policies are being implemented is quite different historically, economically and politically, from other areas in the United Kingdom. These patterns are clearly visible in the sphere of health policy and can be demonstrated in specific changes in mental health laws and services during the 1970s and 1980s. Because the picture is sometimes confused by the fact that policies are not always introduced at the same time as in other parts of Britain, we will look first at developments in England before showing how these have influenced services in Northern Ireland.

Health policies in Britain

Following the re-organization of health and social services in England

117

and Wales during the early 1970s, it soon became clear that some of the problems which had led to this re-organization had been exacerbated rather than solved. Based on the findings of the Royal Commission on the NHS 1976-79 (HMSO 1979) and on Margaret Thatcher's determination to curtail public expenditure, a new healthcare ideology emerged during the 1980s. This ideology stressed: 1) The need for planning mechanisms at all levels of health and personal social services systems – mechanisms which included methods of expenditure control: 2) The need for more effective management systems to ensure efficient use of public resources; and 3) The need to shift the balance of care from institutional care to care in the community. Though all of these policy initiatives affected mental health services, the last one has been the most important. Each change in policy introduced in England and Wales has extended to Northern Ireland either at the same time or a little later. The following time chart summarizes the main developments.

Table 6.1
Health policy initiatives 1974-93

	England and Wales	Northern Ireland
1974		DHSS(NI) Planning Guidelines
1975	'Better Services'	Regional Strategy 1975-82
1976	'Priorities' Document	
	NHS Planning System	
	RAWP introduced	
1978	Strategic Plans: RHAs	
1979	Merrison Report on NHS	
1980		PARR introduced
		'Planning & Monitoring' memo
1981	'Care in the Community '	
1983	'NHS Management' (Griffiths)	Regional Strategy 1983-88
1984	General Management	
	introduced	
1985		General Management in place
1987		Regional Strategy 1987-92
1988	'Community Care' (Griffiths)	
	'Working for Patients'	
1989	'Caring for People'	
1990		'People First'
1991		H&SSBs restructured
		Regional Strategy 1992-97
1993	Community Care co-ordination systems in place	

118

As can be seen from this chart, the mid 1970s saw the introduction of a number of new policies in health and social services to England and Wales. Two of the most important were outlined in the consultative documents: *Priorities for Health and Personal Social Services in England*, published in 1976 (DHSS 1976) and *Joint Care Planning*, outlining a new community care policy, in 1977. (DHSS 1977b) The *Priorities* document, according to Barbara Castle, Secretary of State for Social Services, 'embodied a major new approach to planning'. The need for priority setting was urgent because of the economic limitations outlined in the White Paper on public expenditure. (HMSO 1976) Priorities were suggested for each client group for the years 1975/76 to 1979/80 within an overall growth rate of just over two per cent for current expenditure. (DHSS 1976, para. 11) The need for priority setting was accepted by those involved in service planning but there was dissatisfaction with the financial limitations imposed. (Brown 1977, p. 33) The publication of these documents was followed by the introduction in 1976, of the NHS Planning System in England and Wales and the fixing of health budgets based on the recommendations of the Resource Allocation Working Party (RAWP). (See Ham 1985, Chapter 2)

By the early 1980s both the planning initiative and the community care initiative had gained momentum. The Royal Commission on the NHS had produced its report, highlighting many of the difficulties already voiced by professionals and the public following on the re-organization of health and social services in the early 1970s. (HMSO 1979) The Griffiths report on NHS Management (published in 1983) was promptly acted upon with the introduction of general management into the health services in 1984. The aims were clear – economy, efficiency and effectiveness in all areas of health and social service delivery.

The community care initiative was more difficult to pursue as local authorities were slow to become involved in projects with long term financial commitments. The documents of the 1960s and 1970s had encouraged the use of community based services for some people as a preventive measure or for after care. The emphasis in the documents in the 1980s was different. *Care in the Community* suggested that community care was the best alternative for most people. 'Most people who need long-term care can and should be looked after in the community. This is what most of them want and what those responsible for their care believe to be best.' (DHSS 1981a, para. 1.2) As an incentive, the government was prepared to add six million pounds to existing funds to support the care in the community initiative. (DHSS 1983, para. 6) In 1985/86 the total allocation for joint funding (including care in the community) amounted to £105 million. The purpose of this funding was to enable health authorities to transfer resources for as long as necessary to provide support services for long stay patients moving out of hospital.

In spite of the incentives, progress was slow. The Audit Commissions report of 1986 *Making a Reality of Community Care* was highly critical of developments so far. (HMSO 1986) The government responded to the criticism by appointing Sir Roy Griffiths once again to produce a report – this time on community care. The Griffiths report was published in 1988. His main recommendation – for a Minister responsible for community care, was accepted in principle by the government. However, instead of appointing a separate Minister, responsibility for community care was merely added to the list of duties held by David Mellor, the Minister for Health at the time. The other recommendations in the report formed the basis for the White Paper *Caring for People* published in 1989. (HMSO 1989) This gave local authorities an expanded role in assessing need, designing care packages and establishing links with voluntary and private sector providers of social services. To carry out this role they were expected to establish inspection, monitoring and complaints systems and draw up planning agreements with relevant health authorities, with the specific aim of moving the focus of care from the hospital to the community. On 1 April 1993 the final arrangements to carry this out (including the transfer of funding and changes in structures) were operationalized.

Health policies in Northern Ireland

Strategic planning Though interlinked, management and planning initiatives were introduced separately to Northern Ireland. As early as 1973 the need for the development of suitable planning systems was already recognized. According to the DHSS(NI) report for the period immediately following re-organization of health and social services, 'the changeover to a unified administrative structure provided the opportunity for planning the development of services on an integrated basis.' [DHSS(NI) 1979, para. 2.2] An essential feature of any planning system, according to the DHSS(NI), would be the evolution of a programme of care approach with an interdisciplinary programme-planning team concentrating on the needs of particular client groups. As a first step in this process, the DHSS(NI) formulated and issued to Area Health and Social Services Boards a number of overall objectives and identified certain priorities. This was in January 1974.

In 1975 the first *Regional Strategy* (1972-82) for health and personal social services was published. By 1976 it had become clear that planning for programmes of care was not an easy task. To assist Boards in the development of formal planning structures a DHSS(NI) working group, with representatives from Boards, was appointed to produce 'a simple but practical Guide to Planning'. [DHSS(NI) 1979, para. 2.4] The language used to discuss these planning initiatives reflected that of the consultative document Priorities for Health and Personal Social Services in England published in 1976. (DHSS 1976) In 1979 the DHSS(NI) had to admit that the 'momentum of the planning initiative begun in 1974 had not been maintained.' [DHSS(NI) 1980b, para. 2.2] The NHS Planning System had already been introduced in England and Wales in 1976 where further developments on priority setting resulted in the production by Regional Health Authorities (RHAs) of their first strategic plans in 1978. (DHSS 1977a, para. 1.11)

In March 1980 the DHSS(NI) issued another planning circular – *Planning and Monitoring in the Health and Personal Social Services.* [DHSS(NI) 1980a] This introduced a new planning system designed to ensure the 'most effective use of resources and a more selective approach to the expansion of services and development of facilities'. [DHSS(NI) 1983a, para. 2.1] This document contained a number of guidelines on regional priorities and formed the basis for the first area strategic plans submitted by the four Health and Social Services Boards during 1981. The five year plans, together with yearly operational plans, would form the basis of a five year Regional Strategic Plan. A new era had begun. All future expenditure by each Board would have to be based on stated regional priorities.

During 1980 also, financial resources were distributed to the four Health and Social Services Boards on the basis of Proposals for the Allocation of Revenue Resources (PARR), a report of a working group set up to examine the existing system of allocating resources. The PARR system was similar to the Resource Allocation Working Party (RAWP) formula which had already been introduced in England in 1976. The unique feature of PARR was the inclusion of an additional weighting for the personal social services. [DHSS(NI) 1980b, para. 2.6] Immediately following the introduction of these planning systems a further element was introduced. This was the urgent need for efficiency and economy in the use of decreasing resources. New developments or expansion of existing services would have to be financed mainly from existing resources. Early in 1982, Area Boards were asked to submit proposals for a programme of action designed to achieve efficiency savings and rationalization during the period from 1983 to 1985.

The rhetoric of health services management began to sound more like the business world as the concepts of economic appraisal and efficiency savings became the norm. The Province was still in a favourable position in relation to other areas of the United Kingdom, in spite of the pressure to reduce health and social services spending. Boards were reminded that per capita levels of expenditure on health and personal social services were approximately 30 per cent higher than in England and Wales, and were asked to make efficiency savings of 0.5 per cent per year (as against two per cent in English regions). (Patten 1984) However, Northern Ireland's advantaged position was soon to disappear. In 1985 General Managers were appointed to the four Area Boards, in spite of local opposition. (Community Care, Feb. 21, 1985, pp. 12-14) Districts were re-constituted as units of management, as were large hospitals. Unit General Managers (UGMs) were not appointed at this time as existing structures were regarded as adequate for the task ahead. Apart from the expansion of administrative departments within the hospital sector, these changes did not make a great impact on staff or services. This was due primarily to the fact that levels of funding were still comparatively favourable. Within a year however, it became clear that the management and planning initiatives were expected to achieve rapid results in terms of efficiency savings.

By that time the Regional Strategy for 1987-92 was being prepared. Health and social services in Northern Ireland would no longer be resourced at a higher level than other areas of the United Kingdom. The new strategy was based on a number of financial assumptions: 1) That over the period to 1992 the level of available resources would remain steady in real terms, with just under one per cent a year added to cope with demographic pressures; 2) That cash releasing cost improvements of one per cent per year would generate resources to meet strategic objectives; and 3) That Area Boards should increase their productivity by one per cent per year without any increase in cost. [DHSS(NI) 1986, p. 9] Within these financial limitations each Board was expected to make progress in developing services according to regional priorities.

Another restructuring of the health services took place in 1991. This time the Northern Ireland timetable was in line with England. Unit general managers have been appointed, Health and Social Services Boards have been reconstituted as business organizations, and new lines of responsibility have been opened within Boards and between Boards and the DHSS(NI). The last stage of this restructuring took place in April 1993 with the introduction of new systems for Community Care Management. The new philosopy, incorporating concepts of efficiency and effectiveness, is evident in the *Regional Strategy 1992-97*.

> The strategy identifies eight 'key areas' where specific objectives and targets for improvement are set . . . It is intended that throughout this planning period a concentration on health and social gain, in particular through meeting these objectives and targets, will help

to shift the focus from changes in the management and funding of services to action calculated to achieve real improvements in health and well-being for our population. [DHSS(NI) 1991a, para 22]

Not only are the targets more specific in this plan but the means of monitoring them are clearly spelled out. This is to be carried out by a Management Executive (the Chief Executive and the four Area General Managers) through a Management Plan and Accountability process. (Ibid. para. 27) It remains to be seen whether or not this will achieve the desired aim of improving quality of care or merely result in more paperwork at all levels of the organization.

The community care initiative and mental health policy

The development of community based services for mentally ill people has been one of the priorities in almost all planning documents in Northern Ireland. The first Regional Strategy (1975-82), among eight general objectives, outlined two which were of particular relevance. These were 'the development of community health and social care for the mentally ill' and 'the relief of overcrowding in psychiatric hospitals'. [DHSS(NI) 1983a, p. 25] Mental health services did not feature among the five priority areas in the *Strategy* for the following period (1983-88), although the need for the development of adolescent psychiatry and a medium secure unit for psychiatric patients was acknowledged. The next *Regional Strategy (1987-92)*, contained a very strong statement on priorities in relation to mental health. [DHSS(NI) 1987] One of the three objectives of the strategy was to bring about a shift in the balance of care from institutional care to care in the community, with a planned reduction of 20 per cent in the numbers of people in psychiatric hospitals. (Ibid. pp. 22-24) The latest *Regional Strategy (1992-97)* has mental health as one of its 'target areas of concern', and stresses the need to continue the trend towards a community based service and a further reduction of psychiatric beds by 20 per cent. [DHSS(NI) 1991a, pp. 35 & 46]

The community care initiative in the 1990s is concerned specifically with the transfer of long stay psychiatric patients from hospital to some form of supported care in the community, but the term 'community care' had (and has) very different meanings for different interest groups. (See Jones, Brown and Bradshaw 1983, p. 102) In the report of the Royal Commission on Mental Illness and Mental Deficiency 1954-57, the emphasis was on the provision of services supplementary to hospital treatment. (HMSO 1957) The concept underwent major change in the early 1960s due to the influence of revisionist writing from sociology and within psychiatry itself, highlighting the dangers of institutionalization.

In England the plans of the Ministry of Health during the 1960s reflected this change. During the second half of the 1970s, joint funding arrangements were made to facilitate the movement of patients from hospital to community, as outlined in *Better Services for the Mentally Ill* (HMSO 1975a), although at the time of the Merrison Report (HMSO 1979) some disquiet about the direction of change was being expressed by health professionals and their unions. (Mindout 1979, No. 35, p. 3) In Northern Ireland the integrated structures for health and personal social services made joint funding arrangements for care in the community unnecessary. The development of services for mentally ill people was regarded as a priority in the first planning round after the establishment of the four Area Health and Social Services Boards but the need to move resources from hospital services into community services was not yet on the planning agenda.

Following the publication of *Better Services for the Mentally Ill* the DHSS(NI) appointed a Review Committee to produce a similar policy document for Northern Ireland. Work on this document was postponed pending a departmental survey of psychiatric hospitals and units in the Province. (Donaldson 1979) When the policy document – *The Way Forward* – was finally produced in 1984 it emphasized the themes of the 1960s and 1970s – the need for preventive and after care services in a community framework. It contained little that was different (in policy terms) from the planning circular issued by the DHSS(NI) in 1980. [DHSS(NI) 1980a]

> The department's present policy for the provision of a mental health service ... is to promote mental health and prevent psychiatric illness where possible; to build up services in the community so that the mentally ill may be maintained within their own environment for as long as possible; to provide a range of hospital services so that those requiring in-patient care may obtain that care at the level appropriate to their clinical needs; and to provide an effective rehabilitative service so that patients may return to their own homes and to the community as soon as possible. [DHSS(NI) 1984, para. 2.18)

The Review Committee called for an 'improved range of residential accommodation', closer relationships between statutory agencies to ensure effective use of work placements and between psychiatric hospital services and social services in the provision of day care, and the involvement of the voluntary sector and of volunteers in the 'promotion of mental health education and the development of preventive strategies'. [DHSS(NI) 1984, paras. 4.51 – 4.75] There was no indication in the document that the Review Committee had discussed *Care in the Community*. (DHSS 1981a)

Other documents on community care emanating from England during the 1980s included the *Audit Commission Report* (HMSO 1986), the *Griffiths Report* in 1988 and the White Paper *Caring for People* in 1989 (HMSO 1989). Though they were being studied and discussed in the Province, it was not until 1990 that a policy for Northern Ireland was fully articulated. Richard Needham, Parliamentary Under Secretary of State, in 1989 had outlined plans for community care in the context of the Griffiths report and of government expenditure plans. Though the Griffiths report did not extend to Northern Ireland, there were certain changes which would have to be made in line with government policy as contained in *Caring for People* (HMSO 1989). These changes were outlined in *People First – Community Care in Northern Ireland for the 1990s*, [DHSS(NI) 1990b] The philosophy of *People First* was unambiguous.

It has been said that the best measure of a civilized society is how well it cares for those of its members who for whatever reason cannot live totally independently ... The government's visions of care needed in the community at large has three central principles: first, to help such people to lead, as far as possible, full and independent lives; second, to respond flexibly and sensitively to the needs and wishes of individual people and the relatives and friends who care for them; and third, to concentrate professional skills and public resources on those who need them most. [DHSS(NI) 1990b, p. i]

In order to bring about the shift in the balance of care from the hospital sector a number of changes were proposed. These included: 1) The strengthening of the role of Health and Social Services Boards as co-ordinators, purchasers and quality controllers, relative to their current role as providers : 2) The introduction of systematic assessment methods to ensure proper targeting of resources : 3) The 'full use' of the independent sector in the provision of social services : 4) The extension of Income Support and Housing Benefit to all applicants regardless of their living arrangements i.e. whether they are living in their own homes or in independent sector residential or nursing homes : 5) The establishment of registration and inspection units within Boards to monitor standards in statutory and non-statutory provision : 6) The improvement of planning procedures to focus more clearly on the development, monitoring and evaluation of community care services. [Ibid. para. 1.15]

The themes running through the document were clear – Boards were no longer expected to provide all the necessary services but rather to develop a 'mixed economy of care' making full use of voluntary, not-for-profit and profit making service providers. In order to do this they have

to become experts in monitoring and evaluating services. This is a significant shift in focus – from the direct provision of care to accounting and
inspection. The *Regional Strategy 1992-97* re-affirmed the government
policy for care in the community. In a chapter entitled 'the right care in
the community', the policy was clearly outlined.

> The objective of the Department's policy for community care is to
> provide a range of services that will enable vulnerable people to live
> as full a life as possible, in a setting best suited to their needs – where
> possible in their own homes and communities. Such services must be
> capable of responding flexibly and sensitively to the needs of indi-
> viduals and the relatives and friends who care for them. They should,
> wherever practicable, offer users a range of options. They should
> foster independence and they should concentrate resources on those
> with greatest need.[DHSS(NI) 1991a, p. 26]

In April 1993 the administrative machinery to ensure the success of the
community care initiative was put in place. The impact of this and other
policy changes on mental health services is not yet clear. Before attempting a preliminary evaluation, we will first examine the other major
change which altered the legal context of mental health services in
Northern Ireland.

Mental Health (NI) Order 1986

This Order is an outstanding example of the loss of autonomy in relation
to mental health policy in the twenty year period following the introduction of Direct Rule in the Province. This becomes patently clear when
one examines the answers to the following questions. Where did the
initiative for the change come from? What were the major influences on
the final format? Were there any issues which were publicly contentious
and how were they resolved? What factors were important during the
implementation phase? And finally, what have been the outcomes for
mental health services in Northern Ireland?

Preparation

The Northern Ireland Assembly, set up as part of the process of rolling
devolution initiated in 1981 by the Secretary of State, James Prior, found
its role confined to 'scrutinizing the activities of Northern Ireland departments and commenting on policy decisions referred to it by government.' (Greer 1987. p. 99) It was during the last year of the Assembly's
existence that the Mental Health (NI) Order 1986 came to the statute

books. The impetus for a change in the law had come from England where, since the mid 1970s, there had been a campaign by MIND (Gostin 1975), BASW (1977) and the Royal College of Psychiatrists (1977) to reform the Mental Health Act 1959. The findings of the Butler Committee on Mentally Abnormal Offenders (HMSO 1975c) and the White Paper *Better Services for the Mentally Ill* (HMSO 1975a) formed the basis for discussion. In the *Review of the Mental Health Act 1959* (HMSO 1978) the government outlined proposals for new legislation taking into account the issues raised by consumers and professional groups. After further consultation the Mental Health Act 1983 (for England and Wales) was enacted, followed one year later by the Mental Health (Scotland) Act.

In Northern Ireland it was accepted that it would only be a matter of time before similar legislative change took place. The only people interested in the process were mental health professionals and the two voluntary organizations representing the views of people who would be affected by any changes – the Northern Ireland Association for Mental Health (NIAMH) and MENCAP (NI). For the politicians, mental health was low on the priority list. However, though the impetus for change had come from outside Northern Ireland and though the Parliamentary procedure for public debate on the new legislation was flawed, the Mental Health (NI) Order did receive the attention of the Health and Social Services Committee of the Assembly, a group dedicated to restoring 'some measure of democratic control over the actions of the administration'. (Greer 1987, p. 199) The wish to maintain some local control over legal changes was also strongly expressed by the MacDermott Committee, appointed in 1978 to review mental health legislation in the light of developments in England. [HMSO(NI) 1981] Preparation for the new Order lasted for eight years. Figure 6.1 summarizes the process of consultation and debate which took place during this eight year period.

1975 UK White Paper *Better Services for the Mentally Ill*

1978 NI Review Committee on mental health legislation appointed – the MacDermott Committee (1978-81)

1983 $\downarrow$ ← [UK Mental Health Act (England & Wales)

1984 $\downarrow$ [UK Mental Health (Scotland) Act

1985 NI Draft Mental Health Order prepared by DHSS(NI)

1985 NI Assembly Debate (July)

1986 UK HC Standing Committee (on Statutory Instruments) Debate

1986 NI Mental Health (NI) Order enacted (July)

Figure 6.1 Mental Health (NI) Order 1986 (The preparatory process)

It is evident from this diagram that, though the preparation phase was lengthy, the actual time given to public debate of the Draft Order was very short. It is also evident that the recommendations of the MacDermott Committee were not seen as sufficient mandate for the DHSS(NI) to proceed with the drafting of the Order. Instead the process was interupted to allow for debate and legislative change in England. By the time the Draft Order was published in 1985 the MacDermott Committee was almost forgotten, although some of the issues raised by it surfaced again during the Assembly debate.

The issues

The issues debated most fiercely were 1) The definition of mental disorder; 2) The grounds for compulsory admission to hospital; 3) The scope of the proposed Mental Health Commission; and 4) The involvement of Justices of the Peace (JPs) in compulsory admissions to hospital. Other issues which were discussed, but which did not arouse much controversy, were the need for secure facilities for patients involved in criminal proceedings and concern over the introduction of a holding power for nurses. Two issues which did not feature on the agenda were the role and training of the 'approved social worker' and the 'consent to treatment' section of the new legislation.

The debate on the definition of mental disorder to be included in the new law began with the MacDermott Committee (1978-81) and continued through the Assembly Debate (July 1985) and received its final airing at Westminster in March 1986. The difficulties arose because of differences of opinion as to what should be included in the definition. The MacDermott Committee recommended the inclusion of mental handicap but the exclusion of psychopathic disorder. [HMSO(NI) 1981, pp. 3 & 8] There was no lobby for the inclusion of psychopathy but the inclusion of mental handicap was rejected by MENCAP(NI) and by the British Psychological Socicty (NI Branch) during the consultative process used by the Assembly (NIA 1985a) and again at the committee stage. (HC Deb. 1986, Cols. 1-22) In its final form the Order followed the recommendation of the MacDermott Committee.

The second issue was more controversial. In deciding on the grounds for compulsory admission to hospital the MacDermott Committee based its recommendation on criteria used in Massachusetts, USA. As this recommendation found its way into the legislation in its final form the article is quoted in full here.

> An application for assessment may be made in respect of a patient on the grounds that – a) he is suffering from mental disorder of a nature or degree which warrants his detention in a hospital for

assessment (or assessment followed by medical treatment); and b) failure to so detain him would create a substantial likelihood of serious physical harm to himself or to other persons. [Mental Health (NI) Order 1986, Art. 4(2)]

These criteria reflected the philosophy of the American Civil Liberties Union. This philosophy, attributed to John Stuart Mill's statement on liberty, was made popular in the United Kingdom through the writings of Larry Gostin. (1975, 1978, 1983) According to Mill's statement a man may do what he wills with his own life, provided that he does not cause harm to his fellow citizens. (Mill 1859 quoted in Jones and Fowles 1984, p. 136) The MacDermott Committee, convinced by the American argument that Mill's concept of liberty should apply to people suffering from a mental illness, recommended very specific criteria for compulsory hospitalization. The clause aroused intense opposition during the Assembly debate on the Draft Order. In its written and oral evidence the National Schizophrenia Fellowhip (NI) and the British Psychological Society (NI Branch) called for a return to the wording used in the 1961 NI Act and the 1983 English Act. (NIA 1985a) This would allow for compulsory admission of a patient 'in the interests of his own health or safety or with a view to the protection of other persons.' [Mental Health Act 1983 Sect. 2(2a)]

The objections were based on fear that the enforcement of strict behavioural criteria for compulsory admission might result in extra delay and distress to patients and relatives. The issue was hotly debated at the Health and Social Services Committee and again at the Assembly debate on the Draft Order. The DHSS(NI), surprised at the adverse reaction to the inclusion of a clause which had been strongly recommended by the MacDermott Committee, convinced the Health and Social Services Committee that the underlying principle was important enough to be upheld. This was that mentally ill people should be treated in the same way as physically ill people insofar as this was possible.

As you know, people with a physical illness can refuse treatment; it does not matter if they need the treatment, or if they can benefit from it. Applying the same principle to the mentally disordered, we felt that the mere fact that you could treat a patient and that he would benefit from the treatment, was not in itself a sufficient justification for imposing treatment; there had to be something in addition; and that something is the substantial likelihood of serious physical harm. (NIA 1985a, App. XV, p. 40)

The draft clause, containing the criteria for admission originally proposed by the MacDermott Committee, was approved by the Assembly.

129

The reasoning behind the decision was clearly summarized by Paul Maguire (Alliance Party), a leading civil rights barrister and member of the Health and Social Services Committee.

> I believe that it is an important principle that liberty ought not to be denied, on a compulsory footing, save where there is objective medical evidence of a discernible risk of a compelling kind. The risk of a compelling kind, in my view, must be the risk of physical harm to a person's self or to others.(NIA 1985b, p. 533)

Further issues

Two issues on which there was serious discussion but not a great deal of controversy were on the scope of the Mental Health Commission for Northern Ireland and the role of Justices of the Peace (JPs) in compulsory admission. The responsibility of the commission, according to the MacDermott Committee Report [HMSO(NI) 1981, p. 36] should extend to voluntary as well as detained patients. The committee was interested in the protection of voluntary patients who, because of the nature of their illness, were unable to express volition (referred to by the English MHAC as 'de facto detained'). The debate had been initiated because of the Bickerstaff case – a civil action taken by the EXTERN organization on behalf of a patient who had been transferred to a psychiatric hospital after being admitted to a general hospital. (See NIA 1985b, p. 547) The new Order gave an extremely broad remit to the Mental Health Commission as a result of this debate, making it 'responsible for protecting the rights and welfare of mentally ill and mentally handicapped people living in the community or in hospital'. [MHC (NI) 1990] Nobody questioned the extent of this remit either in the Assembly or Standing Committee debate although it was recognized that the Commission would need to have adequate funding to carry out its task.

The final issue, on which there was some debate but no controversy, was concerned with the involvement of JPs in some admission procedures. The Draft Order had given JPs a role in situations where the nearest relative objected to a compulsory admission. Northern Ireland had not had the judiciary involved in mental health admissions since 1948, so the introduction of a JP at this stage of legislative development seemed a retrograde step to professionals and politicians. As a result of intensive lobbying by the NIAMH and by BASW (NI), the powers were transferred to 'a second approved social worker'. [Mental Health (NI) Order 1986, Art. 5(4)] This is an interesting power. In contrast with the situation in England [Mental Health Act 1983, Sect. 11(4)], the approved social worker in Northern Ireland (in consultation with a second approved social worker) has the power to overrule an objection to a hospital admission by the patient's nearest relative. Of course this power has to be seen in the context of Article 4 of the Northern Ireland Order – compulsory admissions to hospital are for assessment and not for treatment.

The need for secure facilities for patients involved in criminal proceedings or under sentence, was the final issue on which there was a degree of debate. This issue had been high on the agenda before the passing of the Mental Health Act (NI) in 1961 when the NIAMH had lobbied for the establishment of a secure unit in the Province. By 1985 nothing had changed. Patients in need of secure facilities continued to be sent to Carstairs Hospital in Scotland. However, the tone of the debate had changed since 1961. Only the Confederation of Health Services Employees (NI) put forward a case for the establishment of a medium secure unit. (NIA 1985a, App. XI) The Health and Social Services Committee of the Assembly, while acknowledging the problem, was happy to leave the matter in the hands of the DHSS(NI).

> We understand that there has been considerable discussion over many years about the provision of a secure unit but we have been told that doubts have now been cast on whether this is the best way to accommodate patients of this kind. We understand that the matter is once again under active consideration by the Department and we look forward to the outcome. (NIA 1985a, Committee Report, p. 11)

Implementation

The Mental Health (NI) Order 1986, in its final form, differed very little from the first draft. The main differences between it and the 1961 legislation, which it replaced, can be summarized as follows.

1) *Definitions*: Mental disorder is still the general term used, but certain aspects are specifically excluded from the remit of the Order. 'No person shall be treated under this Order as suffering from mental disorder . . . by reason only of personality disorder, promiscuity or other immoral conduct, sexual deviancy or dependence on alcohol or drugs.' [Art. 3(2)] Mental handicap is included within mental disorder and the term 'special care' (introduced in 1948) has been replaced by descriptions of 'impairment' similar to those in the English Act.

2) *Admission procedures*: The 'approved social worker' (ASW) replaces the 'designated welfare officer' [Mental Health Act (NI) 1961, S. 13(1)], as one of the potential applicants for the admission of a patient. The other is the nearest relative as in earlier legislation. The definition of the

nearest relative has been broadened to include someone living with the patient for at least five years and to relatives living in the Republic of Ireland (Art. 32) There are some major differences between compulsory admission procedures in England and Northern Ireland. In Northern Ireland, admission is for assessment only (Art. 4) – not for treatment; the ASW can overrule the objections of the nearest relative after consultation with a second ASW and apply for admission without any judicial intervention [Art. 5(4)]; and the criteria for admission are much narrower than those in the English Act. [Art. 4(2)]

3) *Protection for patients*: The new Order increased the membership and enhanced the powers of the existing Mental Health Review Tribunal. (Art. 70-84) Though all formal (detained) patients had the right to apply to the Tribunal, many did not do so. The new legislation authorized an automatic review every two years for those patients who have not applied for a hearing of their own case. (Art. 73) To further protect patients' rights by ensuring high standards of care and treatment, the new Mental Health Commission has been given wide ranging powers to enquire into any case

> ... where it appears to the Commission that there may be ill-treatment, deficiency in care or treatment, or improper detention in hospital or reception into guardianship of any patient, or where the property of any patient may, by reason of his mental disorder be exposed to loss or damage. [Art. 86(2)]

The remit of the Commission extends to any patient suffering from a mental disorder whether that person is in the community or in hospital.

The implementation of the Act has been uncontroversial. In England, the dispute over the training of 'approved social workers' made national headlines. In Northern Ireland training programmes were implemented without any media attention. The professionalization of the social work role in compulsory admission procedures has raised particular issues about the role of the nearest relative, because in the past most application forms have been signed by relatives and not by social workers. (Prior 1992a) The balance will now inevitably change as the role of the approved social worker develops.

The twelve members of the Mental Health Commission, appointed in May 1986, while aware of their broad remit have focused on specific aspects of this remit. In its first Biennial Report, published in March 1988, the Commission concentrated on treatment plans, consent to treatment procedures and monitoring systems for the management of patients. It also acknowledged the need to monitor the implementation of community care policies, and difficulties being experienced by professionals using the legislation. [MHC(NI) 1988] It is clear from the report that patients were using the opportunities for discussion being offered by the Commissioners during hospital visits and that complaints were indeed being made and investigated. By the time the Commission was preparing its third report in 1991, the changing pattern of care had begun to make an impact. The problems caused by the discharge of large numbers of patients were causing concern. Dwindling patient numbers and low staff morale have not been helped by the gradual run down of hospital buildings caused by the reluctance on the part of managers to spend money on painting and decorating wards which may have to be closed. Surprisingly, the Commission has found no evidence of public disquiet about discharged patients. There have been no shocking disclosures of inadequate care in private residential or nursing homes, and there is no evidence that mentally ill people are featuring more prominently in homelessness figures. (Williamson 1992; HHCRU 1991)

The Mental Health Review Tribunal, set up over twenty years earlier under the Mental Health Act (NI) 1961, has found that since the new legislation more formal (detained) patients are using the appeal system. After an initial surge of interest in 1962-63, the number of appeals settled into a steady pattern of 17 to 20 per year. Applications began to increase somewhat in the early 1980s, but it was only after the passing of the Mental Health (NI) Order in 1986 that there was an upsurge of interest. In the year ending April 1987 there were 55 applications from patients, which corresponded to 33 per cent of formal admissions to psychiatric hospitals for that year. [DHSS(NI) 1987; MHRT (NI) 1992] In 1989/90 the number had increased to 91, of whom 82 were from psychiatric hospitals. In effect, this meant that 40 per cent of all formal (detained) patients in psychiatric hospitals in Northern Ireland during that year requested a hearing of their case. [MHC(NI) 1991, para. 5.1; MHRT(NI) 1992] This reflects a growing consciousness among mentally ill patients and their relatives of their right to question decisions made on their behalf. The increase in applications to the Mental Health Review Tribunal and the willingness of patients to express their views to the Mental Health Comissioners are indications of a trend towards 'user participation' in treatment decisions. However, progress in the development of advocacy systems as envisaged by MIND (Gostin 1975, 1978) and BASW (1977), in the debates leading up to the English Mental Health Act 1983, has been slow. Protection against the possibility of unecessary hospital treatment cannot be provided by legislation alone. It implies the existence of an alternative model of care.

The Mental Health (NI) Order 1986 has made very little impact on the lives of the majority of mentally ill patients – those who are not subject to any compulsory procedures. These are the people who have come to rely on the psychiatric services as an essential support in their lives. In contrast, shrinking hospital services are a source of grave concern to many people, including former psychiatric patients, who wonder about their 'right' to hospital treatment. Mental health legislation can never offer protection from changes in policies. The Mental Health (NI) Order 1986, like its predecessors, did not alter substantially the direction of change already apparent in mental health policy. For the majority of patients, only a real commitment by government to the development of high quality hospital and community based services will make some difference to their lives. As we will see in the next section of this chapter, the community care policies of the late 1980s have had a much greater impact on the direction of service development than the last round of mental health legislation.

Mental health service development

The past two decades have produced a mental health service which will form the basis for that of the next century. This service reflects the changes which have occurred in Northern Ireland since the early 1970s : the change in its political position following the imposition of Direct Rule; the re-organization of the health and personal social services in the 1970s; the introduction of management and planning systems throughout the health services during the 1980s; the reform of mental health legislation in 1986 and the extension of the community care initiative to Northern Ireland in the 1990s

Hospital services

Since 1825, when the first district asylum was opened at Armagh, services for mentally ill people in Northern Ireland have been dominated by hospital inpatient care. In 1961 the number of psychiatric beds available in the Province reached a peak of 6,486 (4.3 per 1,000 population). [HMSO(NI) 1962] The continuing increase in the demand for psychiatric inpatient treatment was part of a trend which had not changed since the early part of the nineteenth century. As hospitals expanded the number of patients also expanded. (See Appendix 1) After 1961 the trend changed in line with other areas of the United Kingdom (although England peaked earlier than Northern Ireland). In spite of the fact that admissions to hospital continued to increase, there has been a steady downward trend in the resident hospital population. Between 1965 and 1983 the number of patients resident in mental illness hospitals fell from over 5,400 to less than 4,000. [DHSS(NI) 1987, para. 4.5]

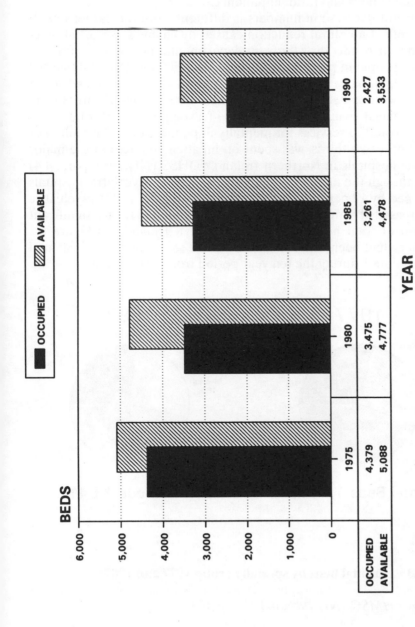

Figure 6.2 Hospital beds (mental illness) 1975-90

Source: *DHSS (NI)*

135

This trend was not a reflection of 'any positive central initiative but rather a number of gradual but continual changes in clinical practice and in admission criteria which combined to reduce inpatient activity.' [DHSS(NI) 1987, para. 4.17] Since then the resident patient population has decreased even further. Figure 6.2 illustrates the downward trend in both available beds and resident patients.

The current decrease in numbers is different from the earlier one. It does not reflect a natural reduction caused by changes in clinical practice. Rather, it results directly from departmental policy to reduce the number of people in psychiatric hospitals to 1,500 by 1997. [DHSS(NI) 1991a, p. 30] Initially this policy was based on cost criteria, as care in hospital is seen as being more costly than other forms of care. In the 1982/83 financial year, out of £39 million (seven per cent of total HPSS budget) devoted to services for mentally ill people, some £26 million of this, or almost two thirds, was spent on inpatient services in the major psychiatric hospitals in Northern Ireland. [DHSS (NI) 1986, para. 4.4) By 1987, though the number of patients resident in psychiatric hospitals had dropped by 12 per cent to 2,911 [DHSS(NI) 1988, p. 20], psychiatric beds decreased at a much slower rate and continued to form a significant proportion of total hospital beds in Northern Ireland. As Figure 6.3 shows, there had been only a two per cent decrease in beds designated for mental illness during the ten year period from 1977 to 1987.

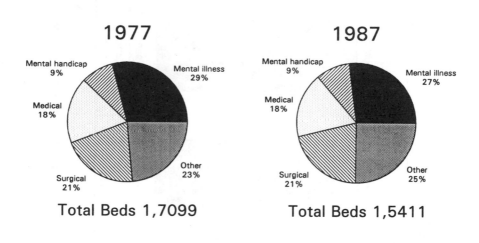

Figure 6.3   Hospital beds by specialty group 1977 and 1987

Source: *HMSO (NI) 1988, p. 19*

By the time the *Regional Strategy* for the period 1987-92 was being prepared, two other developments made it imperative for the four Area Health and Social Services Boards to reduce inpatient costs. The community care initiative and the government expectation that there would be no increase (in real terms) in central funding for new projects meant that there would have to be a real shift in the balance of resources from hospital services to community based services. The financial plan outlined in the *Regional Strategy* called for

> ... substantial changes in the utilization of resources, primarily be transfer of spending from hospitals to community. An annual rate of redeployment of at least one per cent of revenue spending, equivalent to about £28 million in total over five years, will be required ... overall, the proportion of revenue devolved to community services should grow from 26 per cent to around 30 per cent over the planning period. [DHSS(NI) 1987, p. 38]

It was envisaged that in priority areas, such as mental handicap and mental illness, the transfer of resources would be most successful. By 1990, when the DHSS(NI) undertook a review of the *Regional Strategy 1987-92*, it was clear that shifting the balance from hospital care to community care was not easy. Although there has been some increase in the proportion of resources being allocated to community services there was still some way to go to meet the target of 29 per cent. Furthermore, there has been no reduction in the proportion of expenditure on psychiatric inpatient services. In fact it has increased slightly by 0.1 per cent. [DHSS(NI) 1990a]

Because it was recognized that revenue resources, resulting from decreasing bed numbers in longstay hospitals, could not be released immediately, the DHSS(NI) allocated a total of £25 million for schemes aimed at facilitating the discharge of mainly longstay mentally ill, mentally handicapped and some elderly patients during the period 1987 to 1993. [DHSS(NI) 1990b, para. 3.7] The projected costs outlined in the *Regional Strategy* show however, that a downward trend in psychiatric inpatient costs was expected to appear in the early 1990s. [DHSS(NI) 1987, p. 39] Perhaps the planners have underestimated the cost of reducing hospital services. A warning has already come from the PSSRU at Kent:

> ... the experience of schemes to secure the discharge of patients from long-stay wards ... suggests that planners are likely to underestimate the difficulties of implementing them and to overestimate the speed and extent of resource savings and improvement in outcome. (Davies 1987, p. 111)

137

It would be unfair not to acknowledge that, though the changes have not yet affected financial trends, genuine efforts are being made in Northern Ireland to develop community based services. Many of these services were initiated as a result of the funding which has been made available to the Area Health and Social Services Boards to be used specifically for the transfer of patients from hospital into the community. In describing trends in community care services, one of the problems is the fact that there are a number of definitions of what constitutes community care. Does it simply mean the care provided within the statutory sector in hostels and day centres specifically designated for mentally ill clients? Or does it mean a broad spectrum of care – ranging from the informal care provided by family members, through self help groups, to more organized voluntary, private and statutory residential and day care services? If the narrower definition is chosen then statistics are gathered only for specifically targeted statutory services. If the broader definition is used then the difficulty arises as to how statistics can be gathered from such heterogeneous 'providers' of these services. An additional problem arises when one wishes to examine trends in services. The definitions on which the statistics are based may have changed – as is the case in this instance. Notwithstanding these difficulties, some comparisons between services in Northern Ireland and in England during 1990 can be made.

Table 6.2
Mental health services in England and Northern Ireland 1990
(per 100,000 population)

	Northern Ireland	England
Hospital beds available	222	124
Hostel places (staffed & unstaffed)	17	24
Day care places	n/a	15

Source: DHSS(NI)

In 1990 Northern Ireland continued to have a higher ratio of psychiatric beds per head of population than England. The level of provision is due largely to a much higher admission rate in Northern Ireland (an admission rate which is in many ways similar to that in the Republic of Ireland). (O'Hare and Walsh 1985) In 1989 Northern Ireland had a 64 per cent greater admission rate to psychiatric hospitals than England.

[DHSS(NI) 1990b, para. 7.2] Whether these high admission rates are due to the lack of alternative community based services or to other factors, such as the demographic characteristics of the rural areas of Northern Ireland, is not yet clear.

Community based services are extremely difficult to quantify and evaluate. Residential and day care facilities for mentally ill people have been developing slowly and in different ways since the early 1960s. Hostels include a range of accommodation – from highly staffed therapeutic community groups to some virtually unsupervized group homes. Day care ranges from specialized day centres with staff experienced in mental health care, to multi-purpose centres where staff have little or no experience of mental illness. As can be seen from the table above, England had a much higher level of hostel provision (24 per 100,000) in 1990 than did Northern Ireland (17 per 100,000). The English figure represents a 100 per cent increase in hostel provision since 1980. (DOH 1991a, p. 7) The Northern Ireland figure, which in 1990 was 270 places, reflects a decrease in hostel provision over the past 20 years. In 1976, for example, there were 302 such places in the Province, representing 19 per 100,000 of the population. It is not clear why this happened but it is probably related to the fact that before 1990 there was little expansion in private care and no development of voluntary hostels. The situation is changing as the Richmond Fellowship opened four hostels in 1991/92 and plans are underway for further developments by the Northern Ireland Association for Mental Health (NIAMH), by PRAXIS and by other voluntary bodies in co-operation with Health and Social Services Boards. These developments include sheltered housing as well as hostels.

Attempts to quantify day care have also been fraught with difficulty. Day care statistics for Northern Ireland have been omitted from the table above because of the unreliability of some of the available information. With the exception of three day centres specifically designated for mentally ill people in Belfast (Tamar Street, Ravenhill, and Whiterock), all statutory day centres are for mixed client groups. Though no official breakdown of attendances were published at this time the Northern Ireland Association for Mental Health estimated that 697, or 14 per cent, of total attenders at day centres in Northern Ireland in 1982/83 were there because of mental illness. (NIAMH 1984, p. 23) This was the equivalent of approximately 50 places per 100,000 of the population, a figure well below the norm set in *Better Services for the Mentally Ill* (HMSO 1975a), which suggested that there should be 60 day care places per 100,000 of the population. This would give a norm of 930 places for Northern Ireland. The DHSS(NI) set its norms lower than this and planned that 60 places per 100,000 of the population should include both mental illness and mental handicap. In addition to the statutory sector

139

the only large voluntary organization involved in day care services for mentally ill people in the mid 1980s was the Northern Ireland Association for Mental Health which in 1984 had 29 Beacon House clubs with 1180 members. (NIAMH 1984, p. 23) By 1990 the Health and Social Services Boards were under pressure to show that they were providing sufficient day care. Statistics for the year ending March 1990 showed 1,221 mentally ill people attending day care facilities (including adult centres and workshops). [DHSS(NI) 1991b] This would give a ratio of 77 places per 100,000 of the population as against 15 places in England.

Though these statistics cannot be taken at face value, there is no doubt that the community care initiative is being taken seriously and alternative forms of care within the community are being fostered by the Boards in collaboration with housing associations and other voluntary agencies. The 1st April 1993 marked the beginning of a new era in care management, with Care Co-ordinators being employed in the statutory sector to develop creative 'packages of care' to meet the needs of people rather than of organizations, with an emphasis on care in the community. The final outcome of this initiative will not be immediately evident. The target set by the DHSS(NI) in the *Regional Strategy 1987-92,* of a reduction of 20 per cent in the numbers of people resident in psychiatric hospitals, has been met. A further reduction of 35 per cent of beds in psychiatic hospitals is planned. [DHSS(NI) 1991a, pp. 29-31] This will bring the number of beds in psychiatric hospitals in Northern Ireland to 1,500 – its lowest point since the 1870s. It is to be hoped that this will not happen at a cost to patients and their families or carers.

Discussion

During the two decades which followed the very troubled period around 1969, Northern Ireland has undergone major changes in its political position within the United Kingdom and in the administration of public services. The impact of these changes on mental health policies has been highly significant, as many factors arising from general health policies and from the new political context have combined to change some of the basic assumptions which have held sway for most of this century. The assumption that a locally elected government should have control over policies which affect the Province was challenged by the abolition of Stormont in 1972. Under Direct Rule the locus of parliamentary debate on laws or policies affecting Northern Ireland has moved to Westminster. This has resulted in a situation where there is little room for local initiative in policy making, or for the protection of the 'special position' of Northern Ireland in relation to public expenditure.

Because Conservative Government policies during the 1980s were aimed at the reduction of health costs, particularly those incurred in the care and treatment of chronic conditions, mental health services came under particular scrutiny. Northern Ireland was protected from the first onslaught of the cut-backs and maintained a higher level of public expenditure on health and social services until the late 1980s. However, the situation has changed and mental health services in Northern Ireland in the 1990s are subject to the same constraints as those in other parts of the United Kingdom. These constraints include decreasing financial resources; closer monitoring and inspection; targets which include further reduction in hospital services and the expansion of community services; and strict guidelines on future goals. If all of the targets are reached, mental health services in the year 2,000 will show a hospital population of 1,500, a complex mix of community services run primarily outside of the statutory sector, with an increasing shift in public expenditure from hospital to community based services. Whether or not these targets can be achieved and at the same time meet the needs of mentally ill people is not yet known.

Ironically the 'troubles' in Northern Ireland in the late 1960s and the early 1970s left a legacy which should have helped in the development of community services. The removal of welfare services from local government control in 1973 and the consequent integration of health and social services, resulted in an administrative structure eminently suitable for the transfer of resources from hospital to community, and for the speedy implementation of centrally directed policies. The fact that developments in community based services have not been as marked as was expected may be an indication of the consequences of the dominance of the medical model in Health and Social Services Boards in the absence of local government debate on welfare issues. Even if this is so, the probability of a return to local authority controlled welfare services is very low. Equally a return to Parliamentary control from Belfast seems highly unlikely. As social policy in Northern Ireland increasingly converges with that in Britain, it moves farther away from its nearest neighbour – the Republic of Ireland. In 1921 services for mentally ill people in the Province were a reflection of nineteenth century Irish lunacy policies and for that reason were similar to those in the other provinces of Ireland. Seventy years later, while influenced by their origins and by Irish cultural values, these similarities have almost completely disappeared.

7 People and policy

Social policy is ultimately about people who are socially or economically vulnerable. The test, therefore, of the effectiveness of any policy must be the extent to which it protects individuals and their families from exploitation and hardship. The effectiveness of mental health policy is particularly difficult to assess because of the contradictory nature of its social function – sometimes as protection for the individual 'sufferer' and sometimes as protection for society. The following case histories illustrate some of the issues involved in the implementation of mental health policy. The main criterion for selection was the fact that all of these people have been users of mental health services for the past thirty years. All were diagnosed as having a serious mental illness, have experienced admission to hospital on a compulsory basis, and have been the focus for community care policies. These patients were not chosen as a representative sample of psychiatric patients in Northern Ireland.

Gaining access to confidential material is always difficult because of the ethical issues involved. The problem was compounded in this research by the small size of the Northern Ireland population. The accounts are based on casenotes held at the psychiatric hospital to which each patient was admitted most frequently, supplemented by discussions with professionals and (in some instances) with the patients themselves. Names, places and other identifying data have been changed to protect the individuals concerned.

Sheila and Niall

Both Sheila (born 1932) and Niall (born 1924) were diagnosed in the mid 1950s as suffering from 'paranoid schizophrenia'. Sheila was first admitted to a psychiatric hospital at the age of 19. She had been wandering

142

around the countryside 'talking nonsense' and claiming that she had seen a vision of Our Lady in the field near her home. After a short time in hospital she was well enough to go home. However, it was not long before she again became 'bad with her nerves'. Her distraught father wrote to the hospital in 1956.

> I have a Daughter and she is mentally ill this many a year and she has got a lot worse this last 6 months. She imagines everyone is trying to do her harm and she threatens to commit suicide. We have to follow her at night and she is gone away today and we don't know where she is. When she is at home she lies in bed from morning to night and then she rises and would attack everyone with whatever she can get handy, should it be a kettle of boiling water or a chair. It is got impossible to live with her and anything might happen her as she is in a very bad way. Dr Smyth (GP) said to write to you and let you know the way she is, hoping you could take her in for a while as she requires treatment very much. I forgot to tell you she is 23 years of age and her name is Sheila.

Three days later Sheila was admitted to hospital as a 'temporary' patient (compulsory status). In hospital she ranged from being 'dull and withdrawn' to being 'irritable, suspicious and paranoid'. She constantly asked to go home, but her parents refused to have her because of their fear of her violent behaviour. At one stage Sheila had threatened to kill her mother if she got out of hospital. In 1958 Sheila's mental state had not improved and she was certified as being of unsound mind. When the new Mental Health Act (NI) was enacted in 1961, Sheila became a 'formal' patient – a status which she retained until her discharge in 1970.

During the early part of the 1960s Sheila had been allowed home 'on pass' for short periods. However, this was stopped in 1964 as her mother and aunt were 'fed up with her long sessions in bed, her erratic asocial behaviour' and were 'ashamed and afraid of her'. During this time, hospital staff were also finding it difficult to cope with Sheila who had 'poor concentration, poor hygiene' and little interest in any kind of work. Towards the end of the 1960s, in spite of the real possibility of failure, Sheila was persuaded to try living at the newly opened hostel in a nearby town. After moving to the hostel, Sheila got a part-time job doing domestic work. To everybody's surprise, Sheila's employer said she was 'a good worker'. In 1969 she succeeded in getting a fulltime job in a garage – washing cars. Sheila liked the work and (with a lot of help from the hostel staff) managed to look after herself. This was a period of immense progress for Sheila, who though living in a hostel, was still a 'formal' (compulsory) patient of the hospital. This progress was threatened briefly by her family who objected to her working in a car wash saying it was 'rough work – a job for a man'. Fortunately for Sheila, they did not interfere and she continued to live in the hostel and work in the garage for two years. In 1971 Sheila left the hostel to marry Niall, a fellow patient whom she had met during this very positive period in her life. She had only one more admission to hospital (in 1974) and this was after the stillbirth of her second child. After spending 14 years of her adult life as a 'formal' (compulsory) psychiatric patient, Sheila returned to a 'normal' life in the community. However, the story does not end there.

When Sheila met Niall in 1968, he had already been in (psychiatric) hospital nine times. He was first admitted (at age 31) in 1955. At that time he was working as a forester, having failed to complete an agricultural course which he had begun in Dublin. Just before admission he had become moody, unreasonable and inclined to 'rise a row about nothing'. On the day of his admission Niall disappeared after a serious argument at home. Later that day the police were called 'to catch him as he was running through the forest with an axe, calling on Jesus to help him and saying that he saw the Devil out of Hell'. The local priest, whom he knew well, drove him to the hospital.

When in hospital he was 'extremely restless and apprehensive' and refused to allow anyone near his bed, believing an attempt was being made to murder him. He also claimed he could see the Devil. Niall was diagnosed as suffering from 'paranoid schizophrenia' and during his stay in hospital he had a course of modified ECT and later a course of insulin coma therapy. He settled down to some extent but tended to remain 'rather irritable, suspicious and pre-occupied, expressing paranoid ideas'. He was later discharged to his farm which he tried unsuccessfully to run. Niall had eight further admissions between 1955 and 1968. His longest period in hospital was 13 months but it was more usual for him to be discharged within three to four months of admission. Each time he was 'restless and irritable' and had hallucinations which were religious in content. Often it was the priest who persuaded him to go to hospital. He insisted that there was nothing wrong with him, that he should not be in hospital and that he would be all right if he was married. He had made several unsuccessful attempts to secure a wife for himself and blamed the stigma of mental illness for his failure to do so. Because he was obviously lonely, the psychiatric social worker tried to find friendly accommodation for Niall. However, he did not like hostel living or lodgings and before each admission he was usually living alone on his farm or in a small terraced house which he bought after selling his farm.

When Niall met Sheila in 1968 it transformed his life. They married in 1971 with the help of the psychiatric social worker, the community psychiatric nurse (CPN), the warden from Sheila's hostel and the local priest. By this time neither family was interested in the couple's welfare.

Since then (23 years) Niall has been in hospital only four times. Sheila and Niall have two sons whom they raised with intensive support from the psychiatric and social services. The eldest, Andy (born in 1973) was fostered for the first year of his life. The second, Liam (born in 1975) was in care until he was six mainly because of a heart condition. At the time it was decided by the local social services department that the baby would be at risk as Sheila and Niall were only barely able to care for one young child. Liam was allowed home when Andy was four and the family remained on the 'at risk' register.

Niall had very rigid ideas about childrearing and the children had a strict upbringing. Problems which might have arisen due to physical neglect (Sheila did not like housework or cooking) were prevented by placing a Home Help/Family Aid with the family. This woman, who lived locally, worked with the family for 15 years. She helped the children get ready for school every morning and made sure that they had a meal in the evening. The family also had the same social worker for 16 years while the children were growing up. This social worker was instrumental in keeping the children out of care, by being able to reassure social services managers that both children were being monitored and were adequately cared for. He was also constantly involved in solving practical problems in relation to bills, housing and Niall's employment. Sheila never came to terms with household management and her approach to problems was idiosyncratic and usually impractical. For example, her method of dealing with mice in the kitchen was to bring the cooker into the living room and her idea of dealing with an electricity bill was to pray every day that she would win the pools. In addition to the social worker and Home Help the couple had a community psychiatric nurse (CPN) visiting every three weeks as both were on long acting medication.

Sheila is now described as a 'lazy, dirty, overweight' woman who spends every day lying on the sofa, saying 'novenas' (a nine day series of prayers to a favourite saint) and smoking incessantly. Niall is quiet, conscientious, inclined to be over religious and tense. Niall has been in almost continual employment – sometimes on a farm and sometimes in sheltered workshops. Though he came from a 'well to do' family and inherited money in his early adult life, the family have lived in poverty. Niall owned their house and brought home a basic wage, which might have been adequate had Sheila not 'squandered' it on cigarettes and non-essentials. The children always had enough to eat but there was no extra money for luxuries such as school trips or visits to the cinema.

As young children, Andy and Liam accepted their poverty, their father's strictness, their mother's neglect and the constant presence of a Home Help. However, as they progressed through their teenage years, they became more conscious of the differences between their family life and that of their friends. Andy began to stay out late at night and came home drunk a few times. In 1988 both children asked the social worker if they could live in the local Children's Home. Niall and Sheila resisted the idea for a while but as the teenagers became more 'cheeky' and rebellious they finally agreed. Niall and Sheila continue to have the constant support of the community psychiatric nursing (CPN) service. Sheila's last admission to hospital was in 1974 and Niall's in 1988. These are two people with chronic mental illnesses, in a marriage which has always been chaotic, which has been supported constantly by formal structures of care and which has protected them from long term hospital care. Neither of these people could have survived alone.

The issues

One of the most striking features in relation to this couple is the influence of religion on their lives. For both Niall and Sheila it was a feature of their symptoms – Sheila had visions of the Virgin Mary and Niall of the Devil. Both regarded their religious beliefs as central to their lives, a factor which attracted them to each other and formed a common bond throughout their lives. They benefitted from the support of their local parish because of the ongoing interest of the parish priest in their welfare, long after family and friends had abandoned them. The authority of the priest was evident in many of Niall's admissions to hospital. He was often called in by the police or by neighbours to persuade Niall to go into hospital. Religion also dominated family life, with Niall calling everyone for morning prayers and Sheila leading the Rosary every evening.

Another feature of this family's life was the extent to which formal care structures replaced family support and merged with informal networks. Niall and Sheila both lost their family support at the time of their first admissions to hospital. Niall's parents were old and his two brothers had emigrated to America. Sheila's family rejected her completely because of the difficulties they had experienced with her in the years leading up to her committal to hospital. However, throughout their married life they had the support of two people who became increasingly important in their lives. The first was Mrs O'Neill, the Home Help, who lived across the road and who came in twice daily for 15 years – from the time the first child Andy was born until both children went into care. Mrs O'Neill provided the children with a model of motherhood without which they would not have survived. On a practical level she brought some order into an otherwise chaotic household and was a major influence in keeping the children out of care. Austin Taylor, the social worker who visited this family for 16 years, was the other strong supporter of this couple's right to live a normal life in spite of the obvious difficulties.

146

Austin's involvement included premarriage counselling; organizing the wedding; arranging for a Home Help; representing the couple when they were in debt or in trouble with the neighbours and negotiating with the school and with medical services. His final task before moving to another job was to act as mediator in the decision to receive the children into care. The couple also relied heavily on the Community Psychiatric Nurse (CPN) who had called regularly since the time Niall and Sheila were first discharged. Though there were staff changes, it often happened that they had the same nurse visiting for four or five years. In many ways the 'formal carers' became the 'informal carers' for this family. They became their friends and gave the longterm support traditionally provided by family members.

For this couple, 'care in the community' has worked. Sheila began to benefit from 'open door' policies in the 1960s when she moved to a hostel and began working and looking after herself. After three years in the hostel Sheila was able to leave the hospital system completely. However, though both Niall and Sheila made a success of their return to the community, there are important questions to be asked about their way of life. Whose rights were the formal carers protecting – those of Niall and Sheila or those of the children? Have these children been damaged by their upbringing and if so should someone have intervened earlier? Should these children have been kept in care from birth? Or, conversely, would these children have been on the 'at risk' register if their parents had not attended a psychiatrist? The fact that the question of sterilization did not arise, and that the family was supported as a family, reflected Irish rural values. The close monitoring of the family by social services reflected official values – the right of the child to protection from abuse or neglect and the responsibility of the state to intervene in families where there is a possibility of risk. Like other aspects of the life of this family, the issue of the right to parenthood can be viewed from many different perspectives. Perhaps the success or failure of both formal and informal care systems will only become clear as the two children, Andy and Liam, progress through life.

Jane

For Jane, married life was a life full of stress. Born in 1925, she was first admitted to a psychiatric hospital in 1955 showing 'hysterical conversion symptoms due to domestic stress and a recent bereavement'. Her father had just died and she was in constant conflict with her husband whom she accused on this occasion of trying to poison her. Jane was pregnant when she got married at the age of 19. The marriage ceremony was held in the local chapel at six in the morning to avoid social embarrassment. She had eight children in total – six boys and two girls. Between 1955 and 1991 Jane has been admitted to psychiatric hospital care more than 200 times, with early admissions lasting for two to three years and latest admissions lasting only a matter of days. During the 1960s and 1970s Jane was diagnosed as having a schizo-affective disorder. If there was any trouble at home Jane would work herself into a frenzy of anxiety, pack her bag and take a bus to the hospital. It became a battle of wits between her and the consultant in charge of her medical treatment as to how long she was allowed to stay. Jane often said that pregnancy had ruined her life. There was very little anyone could do about this it seemed, as six of her children had already been born before she came into contact with the psychiatric services at the age of 30. Her husband told doctors that he had tried to talk to her about using the 'safe period' but she would not cooperate so there was nothing he could do. She came from a strict Catholic background and would not consider other methods of contraception.

By 1967 (a year in which Jane had 12 admissions) her husband and family were functioning without her, having enlisted the help of her mother-in-law, who lived next door, and her sister, who lived in the same town. Family life was far from ideal. They lived in a two bedroomed terraced house with no bathroom and an outside toilet. Jane told doctors that her illness was due to her intolerable domestic situation, but that her efforts to persuade her husband to move elsewhere failed because he insisted that the family needed the help of his mother. There was constant family bickering, with violence between Jane's husband and their sons and between the couple themselves. Social workers had by then become part of this family network. In 1968, in an attempt to ease the domestic situation Jane accepted a hostel place but the placement lasted only for a few months.

During the 1980s Jane's pattern of monthly admissions was well established. She had become part of the patient community, was known by most of the staff and liked ward life. Her diagnosis was now one of personality disorder or inadequate personality. She no longer showed the extreme symptoms (of anxiety, suspicion and jealousy) of twenty years earlier. In 1982 she was described as 'a very pleasant, easy going and agreeable lady who settled very well into the routine of hospital life'. She also enjoyed the hospital dances and regular Bingo sessions. However, she was 'inclined to be rather lazy and prefers things to be organized for her rather than take the initiative herself'. For a time Jane seemed to improve as she moved into a hostel again and attended a day centre, having by this time totally relinquished any responsibility for her family. The placement did not last and Jane returned home. In 1989

Jane's husband died and she now lives alone. One of her children has been diagnosed as suffering from schizophrenia and two have died of drug overdoses. Another has spent time in prison. All live chaotic lives. Jane continues to use the hospital as a place to escape from the hardships of life. Whenever she cannot cope with any aspect of her life she goes directly there and asks to be admitted.

The issues

This is another family story – this time of a family damaged from the moment it came into existence. In 1944 in rural Ireland an illegimate birth brought with it disgrace and stigma. Jane and her boyfriend had no alternative to marriage. Eleven years later Jane, who was thirty by then, found herself living in appalling housing conditions with her husband and six children. By then she was trapped in a situation over which she had little control. In that year she lost her father who had been her main support since childhood. Since then Jane's life and that of her family have been disrupted continually by her pattern of admissions to hospital. Because she was in hospital so frequently, the family began to function independently of her. She became less important to them and began to feel more at home in hospital. Hospital staff (perhaps unconsciously) colluded with this because she was not a troublesome patient. There seems to have been very little effort to intervene positively in her life to help her solve what she regarded as her two great problems – care of the children and her cramped and inadequate house. The mental health services failed in Jane's case. Not only her own life, but the lives of her husband and children were full of chaos as Jane went back and forth to the hospital. Could any of the damage, especially to the children, have been prevented?

Jane's story can also be viewed in relation to current debates around mental illness in the lives of women. (See Pilowsky et al. 1991) Both marriage and child rearing, though lauded as the most fulfilling female roles in our society, are highly related to mental breakdown in women. (Bebbington et al. 1991b; Paykel 1991) Feminist writers such as Showalter (1987) have demonstrated the role of psychiatry in confirming gender divisions in society by labelling women as abnormal and ill when they reject their roles as wives, daughters or mothers. The hospital often provided an escape route for such women as this label allowed them to be different. Jane's inability to cope with her role as mother of eight children in a two bedroomed house with no bathroom (though they did have an outside lavatory) was accepted only because her protest was expressed in a socially acceptable form – through mental illness. Jane's husband colluded in society's labelling of his wife as mentally ill. He too had been pushed into marriage at a young age. However, as a man, he was free to continue with his social activities. He went to the pub most nights and often went to dances without Jane. He blamed Jane for not being able to control her fertility and made no attempt to change their housing situation. As far as he was concened, Jane was not a good wife nor a good mother, and it was convenient for him to blame this on her illness and not on their domestic situation.

Simon

Simon has been in institutional care since 1953. Born in 1914, Simon lived on the family farm with his mother, sister and brother until the age of 39. He also had another sister and brother, both of whom spent time in psychiatric hospitals. Simon, diagnosed as a 'paranoid schizophrenic', was admitted as a 'temporary' (compulsory) patient in 1953. At that time he was described as 'aggressive and domineering, suspicious and critical of everyone'. Immediately before admission he threatened his mother and sister and attempted to strangle his brother, who was described as delicate and 'simple'. In hospital Simon continued to be restless, aggressive and critical. He regarded himself as highly religious and tended to preach to other patients and staff if given half a chance. In general he did not bother with anyone as he regarded himself as better than the others. In 1955 he was certified under the 1948 legislation. With the change in the law in 1961 he became a 'formal' (compulsory) patient, a status which remained in force until 1978 when he became an 'informal' (voluntary) patient. During the 1970s he was still being described in case notes as 'paranoid, having constant difficulties in his social relationships with other people and shows no insight'.

Though Simon's family did not want him – indeed they were afraid of him – he never lost contact with them or his church community during his stay in hospital, a period of almost forty years. During the 1950s he worked in the shoemaker's department in the hospital and went to the local Baptist church and to his home every week. A letter from his eighty year old mother in 1959 gives some idea of the attitude of the family to him.

> This is a line in regard to the patient Simon P. Smyth my son as he has been coming home to work for a few days every week this last month or six weeks but this last week he has been very cross and irritable and full of worry and he frightened us on Thursday and didn't want to go back to Hospital so will you please keep him in the workshop where he is working at boot repairing as he was content there before he came home and don't let him home for we are not

150

able to work with him and please don't mention our names to him as he is very spiteful and changeable.

After some serious dicussions between Simon and his doctor, he curtailed his visits home for a while. He was master of his own world however and by the 1960s he had settled into a pattern of rising early, washing, eating breakfast and leaving for work, returning in the evening for another wash, some food and a walk before going to bed. His work was sometimes organized by the Industrial Therapy Organisation (ITO) and sometimes through his own church contacts. For example he worked on the roads for the local county council for a number of months. At other times he was employed as a labourer or gardener. He remained arrogant and critical of everyone else and was not well liked by either patients or staff.

In 1969 Simon was taken off medication and offered a place in a hostel. He refused to move to the hostel and continued his pattern of daily activity as before. He had a brief relationship with a female patient who became pregnant. As neither of them wanted the child or a longterm relationship, the baby was adopted. Simon did not have any other friends in the hospital. In 1986 when a survey of longstay patients was carried out with a view to moving some into the community, Simon was found to be eminently suitable for such a move. However, for Simon this was not a simple choice between 'institutional care' and 'community care'. He had already made as much adjustment as he could to community living. He used the hospital as a place to eat and sleep and to keep his bicycle.. His daily life revolved around his church – he did gardening and odd jobs for his fellow church goers and attended services regularly. Simon, seeing no advantage in hostel living, refused to move.

In 1989 (when Simon was 75) he was again approached by staff, this time to see if he would move to a residential home for the elderly. To everyone's surprise he agreed. This was because he knew some of the staff and residents there, as his church choir often sang in this particular home. So, after 36 years in a psychiatric hospital Simon moved out on a trial basis. He had lived there for twenty years without medication or treatment of any kind. When asked what he thought of his new home he said it was fine and that he had no intention of returning to hospital. He is still an eccentric and arrogant man with rigid religious ideas but he is reasonably content and people accept him as he is.

The issues

One of the most striking features of Simon's story is his successful use of the psychiatric hospital as a home. He does not appear to have become institutionalized in the way Goffman (1961) describes it. He did not play a subservient patient role with staff, neither did he make any effort to become part of the patient world. In fact Simon used both formal and informal care structures to make his life comfortable in a way which was different from many other patients. Though his family had rejected him, he continued to visit and to work around the farm when it suited him. His religious beliefs and his participation in a parish community were the major elements in his ability to maintain links with the world outside of the hospital. As the years went by, it became apparent that his family did not want him, that it was highly unlikely that he would marry and that his future lay within the confines of a psychiatric hospital. At the same time, his links with his local Baptist church strengthened. He found meaning in his beliefs and fulfilment in worship. He also found friendship and support among fellow worshippers who invited him into their homes and found him employment. In his move out ot hospital his membership of the church choir made one residential home more acceptable than others. In fact, had it not been for the friendships made through the choir, he might still be in hospital. Regardless of where Simon lives, his identity is clear. As he rides around the town on his bicycle, he is seen not as a psychiatric patient but as a church elder.

In Simon's case, therefore, 'care in the community' takes on an unusual meaning. He did not leave his community though he lived in hospital. In 1986, when efforts were being made to discharge as many patients as possible, Simon did not see any advantage in moving out to a hostel or to sheltered housing. By 1989 he was ready to move, but only to a familiar place where he knew some people. Perhaps there are two lessons to be learned from this – after 35 years in hospital it may take three years or more to complete a move out to the 'community'; and longstay patients (especially older people) are unlikely to want to move from familiar to unfamiliar surroundings. The question remains – was Simon mentally ill or was he merely difficult to live with? Mental health policies in the past have allowed people like Simon to remain in hospital. What will be their fate in the future?

Patrick

For Patrick (born in 1947) there was not the same prospect of institutionalization, primarily because his mother was always willing to take him home. He was first admitted to hospital in 1963, at the age of 14 due to an episode of 'acute behavioural disturbance'. Between that time and 1989 he had 27 admissions. At first he was diagnosed as suffering from 'schizophrenia', presenting symptoms such as 'paranoid delusions of a religious nature and auditory hallucinations'. Later on the diagnosis changed to one of 'manic depression with an underlying personality disorder'. He was still in hospital, as a 'formal' (detained) patient in 1991 with no immediate prospect of discharge. When in good humour, Patrick is charming, outgoing and confident. He makes friends easily and regards himself as a 'lady killer'. However, his behaviour can also be aggressive, manipulative and socially disruptive. He never managed to stay in employment for any length of time though this did not stop him from trying numerous jobs.

One of the most striking features of Patrick's history is the high level of police involvement. In his teens Patrick was often in trouble with the law – initiating fights and damaging property. A number of his admissions were direct transfers from the police station. For example in 1966 he was brought to the hospital by two policemen 'after he had been stopped for riding a bicycle without lights and they discovered it was stolen'. On these occasions Patrick usually avoided being charged or even when charged, he was not given a prison sentence. Patrick's pattern of hospitalization changed after 1982, when his mother died. The time spent in hospital lengthened and the periods between the admissions shortened. Every attempt made to settle him in the community ended in complaints from neighbours and local police. At first he tried to live with an uncle whom he terrorized so persistently that the uncle took out an exclusion order against him. Later, he went to live at a hostel. He was soon asked to leave because 'while there he pinched tea bags, orange juice, and biscuits from other residents, and sold coal from the store'. He also got into constant arguments with the receptionist in the hostel and 'harassed' a female neighbour whose son threatened to beat him up. He alienated himself finally by damaging a television set during an altercation with another resident.

The last attempt to resettle Patrick in the community was an unmitigated disaster. He was allocated a Housing Executive flat in which he lived for four months. During that time he had managed to arouse the neighbours to a frenzy of anger and frustration and to allow the flat to deteriorate into such a state that he was in danger of being evicted for its 'unsanitary condition'. In a letter to the Housing Executive, a neighbour who also happened to be a local politician, outlined the case for moving Patrick out of estate. Patrick had used his flat 'to entertain ladies of varying ages together with groups of young boys'; he had tormented passers by, using abusive language when displeased; women in the area were afraid of him and his flat was smelly to the point of being a health hazard. Because of his antisocial behaviour people of the neighbourhood felt that he was 'not a suitable candidate for rehabilitation in the midst of decent people'.

This and other complaints resulted in Patrick giving up his tenancy and being readmitted to hospital. The admission performed two functions – it provided protection for the community from Patrick, and it also provided protection for Patrick from certain sections of the community. In the locality (as in other similar housing estates in Northern Ireland) any activity which might be construed as damaging the public interest could result in summary punishment by a paramilitary organization. Patrick, by entertaining groups of teenagers had laid himself open to the suspicion of trafficking in illegal drugs. He had also boasted about a sexual relationship with the wife of a paramilitary leader. These activities and his overt aggression towards his neighbours could sooner or later earn him a 'knee-capping' if not a more serious 'punishment-shooting'.

The issues

Patrick is a person for whom the mental hospital has proved to be a real alternative to prison. As a young adult, his aggressive behaviour often got him into trouble with the law. He avoided imprisonment by accepting treatment in hospital and by returning to his mother's home after discharge. The death of his mother in 1982 had a profound affect on Patrick's life. As long as she was alive he always had a home to go to, no matter how aggressive or socially unacceptable his behaviour was. After her death, his uncle tried to provide the same kind of support. However, this support came to an abrupt end when this uncle threw him out because of his threatening behaviour. As an only child with no close relatives, his future now depends on the capacity of the formal care system in the community (hostel or sheltered housing) to contain him. One wonders what this future will be. Will he be allowed to remain in hospital if he wishes to do so? If he is discharged who will be able to cope with his behaviour? Perhaps in the end prison will be the only possibility open to him.

This case illustrates one of the most thorny issues in mental health policy – its function. Are mental health services instruments of social control in society? Who is the law protecting – society or the individual? Is Patrick's behaviour 'bad' or 'mad'. (See Conrad and Schneider 1980) The fact that Patrick was still in hospital in 1991 (on a compulsory order) had more to do with the local community's refusal to tolerate his behaviour than with a medical diagnosis of his illness. Health care staff involved in his life at the time of his last admission to hospital were convinced that his life was in danger from a local paramilitary group. This type of situation often occurs with people such as Patrick, whose behaviour is regarded as a threat to members of a community. Eventually a section of the community will take the law into its own hands and mete out what it considers 'due punishment'.

Mary

Mary worked for thirteen years as a domestic in the psychiatric hospital in which she later received treatment. Her first admission (at the age of 31) in 1969 followed an overdose of sleeping tablets. She believed that 'she was not worthy to be alive and that there would be no rest until she was dead'. Over the next 22 years, Mary had 11 psychiatric admissions as well as innumerable admissions to the casualty department of the local general hospital. Each time she attempted suicide by taking tablets and slashing her wrists or throat with a scissors and each time she telephoned a nurse or social worker before passing out. In the early years, Mary said that she heard voices and felt that people (especially the local police) were trying to harm her. She also admitted to being an alcoholic and an abuser of drugs. At times she spoke openly about what she considered to be at the root of her problems – her lesbianism. She told her social worker in 1972 that she now 'had her sexual desires well under control' and that it was five years 'since she had a relationship with a woman which involved sex'. She knew that 'nothing could be done for her' and she felt hopeless about the whole situation. In 1982 she told her doctor she wanted to die because she was gay and 'nobody accepted gay people'. Mary was diagnosed as having a 'personality disorder with histrionic features'. She had a number of admissions during the 1970s, her longest period in hospital being from 1975 to 1979. According to nursing staff at the time, Mary settled well into the ward and enjoyed hospital life : 'She takes great interest in other people's past and moves from one patient to another collecting all the data possible from them and giving them a run down on her own escapades'. During this time (according to the staff) her concentration was good, she did not look depressed or miserable and there was no evidence of preoccupation or hallucinations. Mary however, insisted that she heard voices and that she felt depressed.

During the 1980s efforts were made to keep Mary out of hospital. Her social worker tried unsuccessfully to get her involved in day care or in sheltered work. Mary was constantly in trouble for being very aggressive to staff or for making advances to the women with whom she worked. As a result of this she found herself at home a lot, which did not help her mental state. At this time she lived with her brother William, who also had a mental illness. Their house was always dirty and chaotic and they had few visitors apart from the commmunity psychiatric nurse (CPN) and the social worker who called regularly. Sometimes William spoke to visitors. At other times 'thinking he was the King of Munster' he merely waved them in and disappeared to the kitchen refusing to give any information. William refused treatment of any kind and at times the responsibility for looking after him weighed heavily on Mary. However, when he died she was very lonely and her suicide attempts increased to one a month. In 1990 Mary was allocated a Housing Executive flat in her local town after her own home was destroyed by a bomb. The community psychiatric nurse (CPN) calls at least twice each week – a preventive measure which has led to a decrease in the number of admissions for attempted suicide. Mary has remained single and defines herself as a schizophrenic who used to be an alcoholic and a drug addict. When asked if she thought there was stigma attached to treatment in a psychiatric hospital she said 'No'. Perhaps for her it had much less of an impact on life than the stigma attached to being gay.

The issues

Like that of Jane, Mary's story illustrates some of the problems experienced by women who do not conform to society's norms and values. While Jane got caught in the traditional female role, Mary did not. Though she had boyfriends as a young girl, she found herself sexually attracted to women. The liberalization of attitudes to sexual behaviour which characterized the 1960s did not permeate to the rural area of Ireland where Mary lived. Her own sense of worthlessness, shown primarily in her efforts to commit suicide, came from her disgust with herself for being 'a lesbian'. Mary did not take on the traditional roles of wife and mother, but neither did she flout society's norms. She preferred to control herself, at great cost to her mental health. At no time during her twenty years of involvement with the mental health services, did any member of staff try to help Mary come to terms with her sexuality. Rather, they dismissed her attempts to articulate her confusion as peripheral to her inability to cope with life. Perhaps this denial reflected social attitudes to the issue of homosexuality, particularly in relation to women. The image of the 'good woman' in rural Ireland allows only for marriage or celibacy.

Mary's case history has two other features which highlight dilemmas in mental health policy. Her brother William, whom she described as 'nutty but harmless', refused any psychiatric intervention in his life. Because his behaviour did not irritate or annoy anyone, he was allowed to live in his deluded world – sometimes as St Francis of Assisi and sometimes as the King of Munster. Mental health services are often narrowly focused on people who threaten society rather than on those requiring care. In planning for new developments, policy makers have to make decisions on how money is going to be spent. Usually, the rights of the wider community to protection from the individual supercedes the rights of the individual to protection and care. Intensive support from the community psychiatric nursing (CPN) service and from social workers has been successful in maintaining Mary in the community. In financial terms, this has been very costly. Will money be available to ensure that discharged patients in future receive similar support?

Common threads

Though these patients had very different life experiences, there are striking similarities in their patterns of illness and treatment. Most significantly, cultural expectations in relation to the individual's life style and family responsibility are clearly visible in the events leading up to admissions and in patterns of discharge. In addition, the importance of the mental hospital as an employer in rural Ireland fostered the development of prolonged informal type relationships between patients and formal carers. Both patients and staff in these case histories have spent most of their lives in a small community. In this way, changes in psychiatric care and treatment have been mediated through a structure which is peculiarly Irish.

The significance of 'the troubles'

The absence from these case histories of life events (deaths and injuries) due to political violence is surprising. Perhaps it is related to the fact that many people affected by this violence do not come into contact with the psychiatric services. Or is it that what we see in the lives of these people is typical of many in Northern Ireland? In the midst of bombings and sectarian killings people go about their daily business as if nothing unusual is happening. Having a job, being married, living in a decent house and being liked by one's neighbours are all more important to the majority of individuals than political issues and sectarian violence.

That is not to say that political events in Northern Ireland have not affected people. They have served to unite people within their religious groupings and have effectively led to the development of segregated public housing and educational institutions. The violence has also been present as part of the backdrop of people's lives. For example, bombing and persecution by paramilitaries formed part of Niall's delusions during the 1970s, Mary had to leave her home in 1989 because it had been destroyed in an attack on the local police station and Patrick was in danger of being punished by a paramilitary group for his antisocial and irresponsible behaviour in the late 1980s. The existence of a guerilla war between the paramilitariies and the security forces has become part of the everyday experience of the people in Northern Ireland. They neither deny its existence nor over emphasize its importance.

157

In reflecting on the lives of the six patients and their families, one is struck by the degree to which certain cultural values not only influence people's lives but determine their patterns of illness. For example, religion played an important role in the lives of all of the patients discussed here. This is hardly surprising in a country where religion forms the basis for many of the political divisions in society. Being a believer has both positive and negative aspects. The local parish priest offered constant support to Sheila and Niall. However, Niall's rigid religious views may have resulted in parenting behaviour which damaged their sons. For Jane, her Catholicism was instrumental in her acceptance of the inevitability of childbearing. She could not conceptualize a life which included birth control, although she was conscious of the damaging effect of pregnancy on her mental state. Being a Baptist was very good for Simon, for whom participation in church activities was a source of support and happiness. For Mary, however, her Church of Ireland community was a constant reminder of her failure to be 'good'. Because she regarded herself as an unworthy person, she no longer went to church, but the values she had absorbed as a child continued to feed into her depression.

For the three women discussed here, the images of womanhood prevalent in their rural communities precluded any deviation from the norms of marriage and family life. Neither Jane or Mary lived up to this image, but instead of confronting the issues involved they escaped into a 'sick role' acceptable to their families and friends. The images of manhood are also clear in these histories. Men were strong and aggressive even in illness. Decisions on money, on housing, on marriage, and on discharge from hospital had always to be negotiated with the men of the family. What emerges from these accounts is that social norms are very stringent in both Catholic and Protestant communities in Northern Ireland and tolerance of social deviance very low. Those who do not conform to social norms are very vulnerable to the label of mental illness, and those who are mentally ill are likely to be highly stigmatized.

Community care networks

When we think of community networks we usually mean family and friends who are not involved in the formal care structure of society. In rural communities in Northern Ireland the boundaries between formal and informal carers are not always clearly drawn. Nurses, social workers, doctors and clergy are often part of the local community within which they work either because they have been born into it or have spent a great deal of their working lives within it. The importance of maintaining links between psychiatric patients and their community of origin is widely accepted as a means of preventing institutionalization and of facilitating discharge from hospital. In these cases we have also seen the importance of formal carers when family care is absent.

For Niall and Sheila the formal care structure, which included a home help, a social worker, a community psychiatric nurse, a general practitioner, a hospital consultant, and a priest, totally replaced the family network which was missing from both of their lives. These people became their friends to whom they could turn on a daily or weekly basis. They merged with the local community as the part of the social context of their lives. For Mary, Jane and Simon, formal carers supplemented and sometimes replaced the support given by family and friends. Without the community psychiatric nurse (CPN) and the social worker, Mary would probably not be alive; Jane used the hospital as a substitute family (with negative effects); and Simon saw both the church and the psychiatric care system as part of his community network.

The stability of the rural community is striking in these accounts, a stablility which shows itself in the patterns of continuity in the formal as well as the informal structures of people's lives. Of course this is changing, as mobility becomes a feature of rural as well as urban life. One wonders if any of the patients who are coming into contact with the psychiatric services in the 1990s will be lucky enough to experience such continuity of care – can we envisage a 'key worker' staying in the same job for ten years?

The effects of policy changes

Four of our patients were admitted before the passing of the Mental Health Act (NI) 1961. Jane, Niall, Sheila and Simon were all 'signed in' by their relatives as compulsory patients – a status they retained for a number of years. In the early 1950s, the pharmaceutical revolution had still not taken place. They received ECT and insulin coma therapy. Life within the hospital improved after 1948 as medical and recreational facilities were expanded. Training for staff, whose number also increased, brought a more enlightened approach to the treatment of patients. The 1960s brought with it the 'open door' policies, the expansion of work projects outside of the hospital, the increase in visits home, plans for hostels and sheltered housing and increased efforts to keep people out of institutions. The new mental health legislation removed certification and the stigma attached to it from the statute books. These policies affected the lives of Simon, Sheila and Jane in different ways. Simon, instead of working in the hospital shoemaker's department, was employed by the local council to work on the roads. He bought a bicycle and used it to visit home and to go to church. Sheila began work as a domestic in a private house, travelling out of the hospital each day in the minibus bought by the occupational therapy department for patients willing to try working outside of the hospital. Jane by this time was becoming institutionalized, making friends among both patients and staff and enjoying ward life. The battle by the medical staff to prevent her from making the hospital her home began. Her periods in hospital were shortened from years to months and some effort was made to involve her husband in dealing with her problems. Their efforts were not successful but perhaps it represented some progress as in an earlier era Jane would probably have been allowed to stay in hospital.

The expansion of psychiatric services to support patients in the community, particularly the community psychiatric nursing service and hospital based social work service made a return to the community possible for some patients and more comfortable for others. For Niall and Sheila these services were an essential part of their lives, making marriage and child rearing possible. For Mary it has been the difference between life and death. It is not yet clear how the decarceration policies of the 1990s will work. For patients such as Simon who have been moved to another institution there will be few problems. However, it is not so easy to predict what will happen to someone like Patrick who has no family, who cannot cope with independent living and whose anti-social behaviour may lead him into trouble. Will the hospital continue to provide a place for him to live? What is evident is that the psychiatric hospital has been many things to many people. The provision of treatment for mental illness has been part but by no means all of its social function. If this function is to change then the tasks which it performed in the past will no doubt be transferred to other organizations in the future.

8 A final word

In looking back at almost a century of mental health policy, a number of themes emerge which highlight some of the dilemmas involved in planning health and social services in a context dominated by other concerns. Some of these themes are familiar to students of social policy in Northern Ireland and some are new. The most important can be summarized as follows :

1 Changes in mental health policy have been determined largely by the political context.

2 Special factors in Northern Ireland have often not been recognized in policy planning and implementation.

3 The expansion and contraction of mental health service provision has had little to do with need.

Politics and mental health policy

The importance of political factors in the development of mental health policy has been demonstrated throughout this study. Though sociological and economic explanations are important in helping our understanding of the composition of the patient population in hospital and of the impact of certain policies on this population, the main influences on the direction of change in the services have not been social or economic – they have been political. Two current debates are relevant to this area of study.

Parity and devolution The Northern Ireland government prior to 1972 either followed parity with Britain or used its devolved powers to do things differently. (Birrell 1990, p. 7) Certain areas of policy such as health and social security have followed the parity principle, while education, personal social services and housing have been substantially different. Most writers agree that since 1972, when Direct Rule was introduced, the pressure for uniformity with Britain has increased. (See Connolly and Loughlin 1990; Birrell 1990; Ditch and Morissey 1992) Between 1921 and 1932, and again between 1948 and 1959, there were significant differences in mental health legislation between Northern Ireland and Britain. At all other times policies (including legislation) have paralleled Britain. However, the question of parity is not a simple one. As Birrell and Murie (1980, p. 280) point out, it can mean uniformity, similarity in most respects, or similarity only in the broadest terms and there is also the distinction between parity as input, as output or as outcome. (Ditch 1984) In relation to mental health, increased expenditure on hospital services during the 1950s was aimed at achieving parity of outputs and of outcomes. However, there was still room for innovation. Since 1973 the trend toward 'similarity in most respects' is clear in mental health policy and legislation, a trend which reflects the movement towards convergence between Northern Ireland and Britain.

Political conflict and social policy The changing and often unstable political context in Northern Ireland has provided a policy environment dominated by the constitutional question.

> Whereas in Britain the basic political division is one of social and class issues – labour versus capital – in Northern Ireland it is primarily concerned with the constitutional question: Should Northern Ireland remain part of the United Kingdom or become part of a United Ireland? (Connolly and Loughlin 1990, p. 5)

The civil unrest spawned by this question has had varying effects on different social policies. Housing policy, for example, is one of the areas which has been profoundly and demonstrably affected. However, the relationship between violence and mental health policy is more difficult to quantify and findings from studies on the impact of civil unrest have been inconclusive. Some of the problems are methodological. Mental health statistics in themselves do not contain the answers. Neither do general surveys on perceptions of violence. The only conclusion to be drawn from the current research is that for the majority of the population it is safer (from a mental health point of view) to deny the reality of the risks involved in living in a situation of violence, than to allow oneself to worry about it. However, though there are no definitive answers on the impact of the 'troubles' on the mental health of individuals, it is clear that services and legislation were shaped by the impact of the political crisis which has continued since the late 1960s.

162

Northern Ireland is different

Even within Northern Ireland it is often assumed that health policies can be transferred directly from Britain. However, this has often led to unexpected consequences both in the interpretation and implementation of these policies. The most obvious features which make the Province different from other parts of the United Kingdom are the relative social and economic disadvantage of the region, the dominance of central government in social service provision and the existence of cultural and historical links with the Republic of Ireland.

Northern Ireland as a disadvantaged region By a number of indicators, such as high unemployment, high dependency on social security, high rates of infant and perinatal mortality and high cost of living, Northern Ireland is more disadvantaged than any other region of the United Kingdom. (Evason et al. 1976; Darby and Williamson 1978; Ditch and Morrissey 1992) Since the 1970s, in an attempt to offset the disadvantages, there has been a consistent pattern of higher public expenditure in the Province than in any other area of the United Kingdom. Whether this expenditure is based on the principles of equity (because of greater needs) or on those of social order (to prevent outbursts of violence) does not affect the outcome of this ongoing injection of funds into all public services. Health services have expanded and flourished. Until the late 1980s, these services were protected from Conservative government cutbacks which had been imposed earlier in the decade on health and social services expenditure in Britain. Now, however, there is no such protection, in spite of the fact that the link between deprivation and mental illness has been proven many times. (Belle 1990; Bebbington et al. 1991a; Thornicroft 1991: Reissman et al. 1964)

The dominance of central government in the planning and delivery of social services One of the outcomes of the political violence in the 1960s was the decision by Westminster to impose Direct Rule in 1972 and to pursue policies which would redress the balance of discrimination which had prevailed against the Catholic minority. Direct Rule and the removal of education, housing, health and welfare from local authority control have led to a significant difference in the balance of power among policy making bodies. As the influence of local government and the involvement of local politicians in the policy network have decreased, the role of central government, supported by a strong civil service, has increased. One of the results of these developments has been the removal of all responsibilities for health and social services from local government control and the integration of these services under Area Health and

Social Services Boards. This integration may have provided a more favourable context for the development of community based mental health services but it has also removed the debate on the value of local control over local services, a debate which has led to many innovative local authority projects in England, Wales and Scotland.

An important aspect of the shift in the balance of power from local to central authorities and from elected representatives to civil servants, has been the increase in bureaucratic control over policy making and implementation. With the exception of debates spawned by preparations for changes in mental health laws, there has been no debate on mental health issues in the Province. This has meant that the implementation of new laws and policies have been determined primarily by health service administrators both at central and local level. The lact of local debate is particularly relevant in mental health matters where the consumers of the services are often unable to master the socially accepted means of public lobbying. As the numbers of beds in psychiatric hospitals decrease, who will ensure that community services provide an adequate replacement?

Links with the Republic of Ireland The fact that Northern Ireland is geographically part of Ireland is often overlooked because of the divergence in laws and social policies since 1921. However, in relation to mental health services the legacy of the past has been very influential in determining many aspects of policy implementation. Patterns of hospitalization were established by the building of six asylums as part of a network of district asylums in nineteenth century Ireland. Before the Second World War many aspects of public policy in Northern Ireland continued to be influenced by developments in Dublin with the Mental Health Act (NI) 1948 being the last example of this influence on mental health policy. What remains is not only a legacy from the past in terms of mental health provision, but a reflection of current cultural similarities between the two parts of Ireland. For example, statistical patterns of mental hospital admission and discharge have more in common with each other than either has with the United Kingdom. However, because of the ever increasing divergence in policies, there is very little common ground for a comparative debate between mental health professionals or planners on both sides of the Border. This seems to be a waste of a valuable resource for all concerned.

No evidence of a 'needs led' service

As mental hospital beds continue to shrink from a high of 6,500 in 1961 to a projected low of 1,500 in 1997, one wonders what this means in terms of the prevalence of mental disorder in Northern Ireland or the adequacy of current provision? Does it mean that mental illness is truly a myth – that society no longer needs to confine its deviants to institutions in order to control them? Have we as a society become more humane in our attitude to those who behave 'differently'? Or is Andrew Scull (1984) right in interpreting the official reduction of state provision for mental disorder as meeting the needs of our capitalist economy? This research has shown that neither of these interpretations can be taken as explanatory. The expansion of the mental hospital system in Northern Ireland before the 1960s has to be understood in the light of extra health service funding after 1948 and efforts to destigmatize psychiatric treatment by encouraging people to use the mental hospital as they would a general hospital. The current contraction of hospital beds is also related to funding – or rather the lack of it. What is worrying is the continued high rate of expenditure on hospital services in spite of decreasing patient numbers. It will take some time to dismantle a system which is of undoubted benefit to people employed as health administrators and professionals – much longer than it has taken to discharge patients. The question arises: who needs the hospitals most – the staff or the patients? Some patients regarded as 'legitimate' targets for psychiatric treatment during the 1970s are now being discharged to their families and communities. Have they been cured or were they ever ill?

As more people are discharged from hospital the burden of care moves from the statutory to the voluntary and informal care sectors. Government expenditure on health services is highly visible. Private expenditure (particularly in the context of families or friends) is almost invisible. As the care of potential and former patients moves from the publicly funded hospital system will it also move out of the realm of public responsibility? In Northern Ireland, the Area Health and Social Services Boards are theoretically committed to monitoring and evaluating the effects of current community care policies, in order to ensure that cut backs in central government expenditure on health do not necessarily lead to hardship among people who, until recently, were cared for within the statutory system. (See HHCRU 1991) However, as this study has demonstrated, the power of Area Boards is dwindling steadily in the face of health policies emanating from England. The convergence of policy between England and Northern Ireland, which has accelerated during the late 1980s, is an example of the far reaching inhibiting effect of the current form of government (Direct Rule) on every aspect of social policy. The combination of strong central control with a local government structure which has no control over social services, housing or education, has left Northern Ireland with no forum for debate and very little room for local initiative.

The problem is intensified by difficulties in defining need. Official mental health statistics tell us little about the existence of mental illness. Statistics can be highly informative if used to help us understand how and why people suffer from different forms of mental disorder. Research has shown the vulnerability of certain groups, including married women, people living alone, immigrants and poor people. However, this kind of statistical research is not useful to a government trying to prove a decreasing need for costly services. Current mental health statistics focus on throughput, bed usage and staff patient ratios to ensure the best use of public funds.

For people suffering from mental illness and for their carers, this is a very worrying time. Mental health policy in the 1990s is undergoing the kind of change of direction which has been paralleled only by that which took place in the 1820s, when district asylums were first built in Ireland. The rise and fall of the asylum as the central focus of treatment for mental illness is now history. The focus for care and treatment is firmly back in the family and community. The Irish are known throughout the world for their friendliness and family loyalty. Only time will tell if this positive attitude extends to the care of the more vulnerable members of society.

Appendix 1

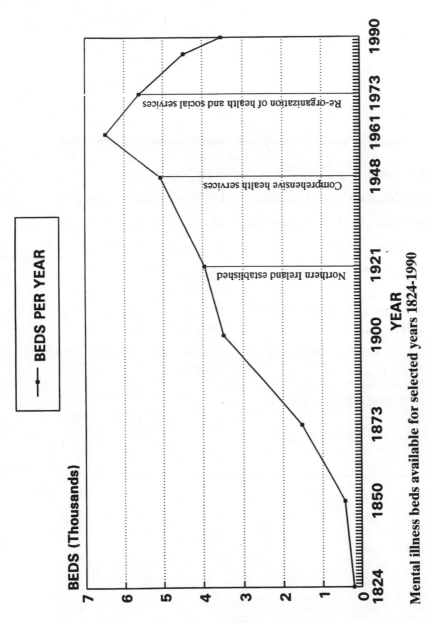

BEDS (Thousands)

BEDS PER YEAR

Northern Ireland established

Comprehensive health services

Re-organization of health and social services

1824 1850 1873 1900 1921 1948 1961 1973 1990

YEAR

Mental illness beds available for selected years 1824-1990

Source: *Government Statistics*

Appendix 2

Names of mental hospitals in Northern Ireland after 1948

Former Name	New Name
Antrim County Mental Hospital	Holywell Hospital, Antrim
Armagh County Mental Hospital	St Lukes's Hospital, Armagh
Belfast Mental Hospital	Purdysburn Hospital, Belfast
Downpatrick Mental Hospital	Downshire Hospital, Downpatrick
Londonderry City and County Mental Hospital	Londonderry and Gransha Hospital, Londonderry
Tyrone and Fermanagh Mental Hospital	Tyrone and Fermanagh Hospital, Omagh

Source: HMSO(NI) 1951, p. 80

Appendix 3

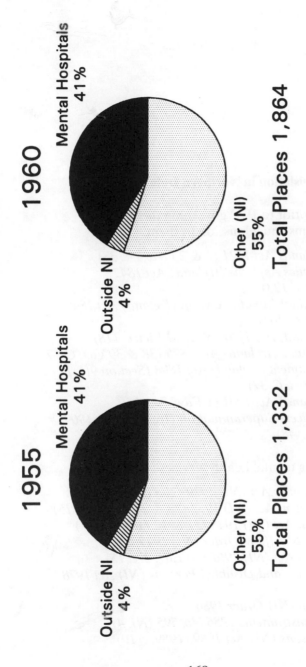

1960

Mental Hospitals
41%

Outside NI
4%

Other (NI)
55%

Total Places 1,864

1955

Mental Hospitals
41%

Outside NI
4%

Other (NI)
55%

Total Places 1,332

Special care patients in residential accommodation 1955 and 1960

Source: *NIHA 1955 & 1960*

Appendix 4

Mental health legislation in Northern Ireland

Statutes in force prior to 1932 governing the provision
of asylums and admission to them:

Lunacy (Ireland) Act 1821 (1 & 2 Geo. 4. c. 33)
Private Lunatics Asylums (Ireland) Act 1842
(5 & 6 Vict. c. 123)
Central Criminal Lunatic Asylum (Ireland) Act 1845
(8 & 9 Vict. C. 107)
Lunacy (Ireland) Act 1867 (30 & 31 Vict. c. 118)
Lunatic Asylums (Ireland) Act 1875 (38 & 39 Vict. C. 67)
Local Government (Ireland) Act 1898 [Section 9(6)]
(61 & 62 Vict. C. 37)
Lunacy (Ireland) Act 1901 (1 Edw. 7. c. 17)
Asylums Officers Superannuation (Ireland) Act 1909
(9 Edw. 7. c. 48)

Statutes governing mental health services since 1932:

Criminal Lunatics Act (NI) 1929 (20 Geo. 5. c. 19)
Mental Treatment Act (NI) 1932 (22 & 23 Geo. 5. c. 15)
Mental Health Act (NI) 1948 (11 & 12 Geo 6. c. 17)
Mental Patients' Affairs Order (NI) 1949
Mental Health Act (NI) 1961 (10 Eliz. 2. c. 15)
Chronically Sick and Disabled Persons (NI) Act 1978
(1978, c. 53)
Mental Health (NI) Order 1986
[Statutory Instruments 1986 No. 595 (NI. 4)]
Disabled Persons (NI) Act 1989 (1989, c. 10)

Bibliography

Abel-Smith, Brian (1957) *Finance of the Health Services.* Paper given at the Northern Ireland Health Services Conference.

Abel-Smith, B. and Titmuss, R. M. (1956) *The cost of the National Health Services in England and Wales.* Cambridge: University Press.

Abraham, George Whitley (1886) *The Law and Practice of Lunacy in Ireland.* Dublin: Ponsonby.

Adams, G. F. and Cheeseman, E. A. (1951) *Old People in Northern Ireland.* Belfast: NIHA.

Alexander, Franz and Selesnick, Sheldon (1966) *The History of Psychiatry.* New York: Mentor Books.

Anderson-Ford, David and Halsey, Michael (1984) *Mental Health: Law and Practice for Social Workers.* London: Butterworths.

Armagh (1948) *Armagh Mental Hospital Annual Report for 1948.*

Arthur, Paul (1980) *Government and Politics of Northern Ireland* Essex: Longman.

Baldwin, S. (1985) *The Costs of Caring.* London: Routledge and Kegan Paul.

Banton, R., Clifford, P. et alia (1985) *The Politics of Mental Health.* London: Macmillan Ltd.

Barnes, M., Bowl, R., and Fisher, M. (1990) *Sectioned: Social Services and the 1983 Mental Health Act.* London: Routledge.

Barton, W. R. (1959) *Institutional Neurosis.* Bristol: John Wright and Sons.

Barrington, Ruth (1987) *Health Medicine and Politics in Ireland 1900-70.* Dublin: Institute of Public Administration.

BASW (1977) *Mental Health Crisis Services – A New Philosophy: Report of evidence of BASW on the Review of the Mental Health Act 1959.* Birmingham: BASW.

Bean, Philip (1980) *Compulsory Admissions to Mental Hospitals.* London: John Wiley and Sons.

Bean, Philip (ed.) (1983) *Mental Illness: Changes and Trends.* London: John Wiley and Sons.

Bean, Philip (1986) *Mental Disorder and Legal Control.* Cambridge: Cambridge University Press.

Bebbington, P. E., Tennant, C. and Hurry, J. (1991a) 'Adversity in groups with an increased risk of minor affective disorder'. *British Journal of Psychiatry.* Vol. 158. pp. 33-40.

Bebbington, P. E., Dean, C., Der, G., Hurry, J., and Tennant, C. (1991b) 'Gender, parity and the prevalence of minor affective disorder'. *British Journal of Psychiatry.* Vol. 158. pp. 40-45.

Bell. Dr. (1968) 'The Child Guidance Service in Northern Ireland'. *Internal Report for the Ministry of Health and Social Services (NI).* Belfast: Min. H&SS.

Bell, P. N. (1987) 'Direct Rule in Northern Ireland' in R. Rose (ed) *Ministers and Ministries: A functional analysis.* Ch. 7. Oxford: Clarendon Press.

Belle, D. (1990) 'Poverty and women's mental health'. *American Psychologist.* Vol. 45. No. 3. pp. 385-89.

Berrios, G. E. (1991) 'Psychosurgery in Britain and elsewhere: a conceptual history' in Berrios, G. and Freeman, H. (eds) pp. 180-96.

Berrios, G. and Freeman, H. (eds) (1991) *150 Years of British Psychiatry 1841-1991.* London: Gaskell and Royal College of Psychiatrists.

Bew, Paul. Gibbon, Peter and Patterson, Henry (1979) *The State in Northern Ireland 1921-72.* Manchester: Manchester University Press.

Birrell, Derek (1990) 'The Development of Social Administration'. *Paper delivered at the University of Ulster at Coleraine in October.* (Unpublished)

Birrell, Derek and Murie, Alan (1975) 'Ideology, Conflict and Social Policy'. *Journal of Social Policy.* Vol. 4. No. 3. pp. 243-58.

Birrell, Derek and Murie, Alan (1980) *Policy and Government in Northern Ireland.* Dublin: Gill and Macmillan.

Birrell, Derek and Williamson, Arthur (1983) 'Northern Ireland's Integrated Health and Personal Social Service Structure' in A. Williamson and G. Room (eds) *Health and Welfare States of Britain.* pp. 130-50. London: Heinemann.

Blake, John W. (1956) *Northern Ireland in the Second World War.* Belfast: HMSO.

Bluglass, R. (1983) *A Guide to the Mental Health Act 1983.* Edinburgh: Churchill Livingstone.

Booz, Allen and Hamilton (1972), *Summary of report on the re-organization of Health and Social Services in Northern Ireland.* Belfast: HMSO.

Bradshaw, Jonathan (1989) *Social Security Parity in Northern Ireland.* Belfast: Policy Research Institute (PRI).

Brown, Muriel (1977) 'Priorities for Health and Social Services', in K. Jones (ed) *The Yearbook of Social Policy in Britain 1976.* pp. 21-34. London: Routledge and Kegan Paul.

Brown, Phil (ed) (1985) *Mental Health Care and Social Policy.* Boston: Routledge and Kegan Paul.

Brown, R. (1987) *The Approved Social Worker's Guide to the Mental Health Act 1983.* London: Reed Publishing. (First published 1983)

Buckland, Patrick (1979) *The Factory of Grievances: Devolved Government in Northern Ireland 1921-39.* Dublin: Gill and Macmillan.

Buckland, Patrick (1981) *A History of Northern Ireland.* Dublin: Gill and Macmillan.

Burke, Helen (1987) *People and the Poor Law in nineteenth century Ireland.* West Sussex: Women's Education Bureau.

Burton, Mark (1983) 'Understanding mental health services: Theory and Practice'. *Critical Social Policy.* Vol.3. No.7. pp. 54-74.

Burton, Robert (1621) *The Anatomy of Melancholy.* 6th edition: edited by Floyd Dell and Paul Jordan-Smith (1927). New York: Tudor Publishing Company.

Busfield, Joan (1986) *Managing Madness: Changing Ideas and Practice.* London: Hutchinson.

Butler, Tom (1985) *Mental Health, Social Policy and the Law.* London: Macmillan Press Ltd.

Bynum, W. F. Porter, R. and Shepherd, M. (eds) (1985a) *The Anatomy of Madness.* Vol. 1. London: Tavistock.

Bynum, W. F. Porter, R. and Shepherd, M. (eds) (1985b) *The Anatomy of Madness.* Vol. 2. London: Tavistock.

Cairns, Ed and Wilson, Ronnie (1984) 'The impact of Political Violence on Mild Psychiatric Morbidity in Northern Ireland'. *British Journal of Psychiatry.* Vol. 145. pp. 631-35.

Cairns, Ed and Wilson, Ronnie (1989) 'Mental Health Aspects of Political Violence in Northern Ireland'. *Int. J. Ment. Health.* Vol. 18. No. 1. pp. 38-56.

Cassin, P. J. (1934) 'Lunacy Certification in Ireland'. *Irish Journal of Medical Science.* January. pp. 22-27.

Clare, Anthony (1976) *Psychiatry in Dissent.* London: Tavistock.

Cohen, Stanley and Scull, Andrew (eds) (1983) *Social Control and the State Historical and Comparative Essays.* Oxford: Martin Robertson.

Coleman, S., Wilson, R., (1991) 'Psychiatric and social characteristics of homeless hostel residents in Northern Ireland'. *Irish Journal of Psychology.* Vol. 12. No. 3. pp. 316-24.

Colles, J. M. (circa 1890) *The Lunacy Act and Orders – with forms and the County Court Act and Rules.* Dublin: William Mc Gee (Also London: Stevens and Haynes). (2nd edition – no date)

Connolly, Michael (1985) 'Has integration worked: The Health and Personal Social Services in Northern Ireland?'. *Health Care UK.* pp. 89-91. London: CIPFA.

Connolly, M. E., and Loughlin, S. (eds) (1990) *Public Policy inNorthern Ireland: Adoption or Adaptation.* Belfast: Policy Research Institute (PRI).

Conrad, Peter and Schneider, Joseph (1980) *Deviance and Medicalisation – from Badness to Sickness.* St. Louis: C. V. Mosby Co.

Curran, Peter (1988) 'Psychiatric Aspects of Terrorist Violence: Northern Ireland 1969-87'. *British Journal of Psychiatry.* Vol. 153. pp. 470-75.

Curran, P., Bell, P., Murray, G., Loughrey. G., Roddy, R. and Rocke. L. G. (1990) 'Psychological Consequences of the Enniskillen Bombing'. *British Journal of Psychiatry.* Vol. 156. pp. 479-82.

Darby, John (ed) (1983), *Northern Ireland: The Background to the Conflict.* Belfast: Appletree Press.

Darby, John and Williamson, Arthur (eds) (1978) *Violence and the Social Services in Northern Ireland.* London: Heinemann.

Davies, B. (1984) 'The Community Care Approach: present policies and future strategies'. Kent: University, PSSRU Paper 363.

Davies, B. (1987) 'Plans for the Health and Personal Social Services in Northern Ireland'. Kent: University, PSSRU Paper 434.

Davies, B. P. and Challis, D. (1986) *Matching Resources to Needs in Community Care.* Aldershot: Gower.

Dear, Michael and Wolch, Jennifer (1987) *Landscapes of Despair: From de-institutionalisation to homelessness.* Cambridge: Polity Press.

Deutsch, Albert (1937) *The Mentally Ill in America.* Columbia: University Press.

DHSS (1963) *Health and Welfare – The Development of Community Care: Plans for the health and welfare services of the local authorities in England and Wales.* Cmnd. 1973. London: HMSO.

DIISS (1970) *National Health Service – The future structure of the NHS.* Green Paper. London: HMSO.

DHSS (1976) *Priorities for the Health and Personal Social Services in England – A consultative document.* London: HMSO.

DHSS (1977a) *Priorities in the Health and Personal Social Services – The Way Forward.* (Further discussion of the Government's national strategy based on the consultative document 'Priorities in the Health and Personal Social Services'). London: HMSO. (September)

DHSS (1977b) Document on *Joint Care Planning between Health and Local Authorities.* Circular HC (77) 17, LAC (7710). London: HMSO.

DHSS (1978) *Review of the Mental Health Act 1959.* Cmnd. 7320. London: HMSO.

DHSS (1979) *Patients First – A consultative paper on the structure and management of the NHS in England and Wales.* London: HMSO. (December)

DHSS (1980) *Organisational and Management Problems of Mental Illness Hospitals* (The Nodder Report). London: HMSO.

DHSS (1981a) *Care in the Community – A consultative document on moving resources for care in England.* London: HMSO. (July)

DHSS (1981b) *Care in Action – A handbook of policies and priorities for the Health and Personal Social Services in England.* London: HMSO.

DHSS (1981c) *Report of a Study on Community Care.* London: HMSO.

DHSS (1983) *Explanatory notes on 'Care in the Community'.* London: HMSO.

DHSS (1986) *The Health Service in England : Annual Report 1985-86.* London: HMSO. (December)

DHSS(NI) (1975) *Strategy for the development of Health and Personal Social Services in Northern Ireland.* Belfast: HMSO.

DHSS(NI) (1979) *Report on the Administration of the Health and Social Services in Northern Ireland 1 Oct 1973-31 Dec 1976.* Belfast: HMSO.

DHSS(NI) (1980a) *Planning and Monitoring in the Health and Personal Social Services.* HSS(P) 1/80. Belfast: DHSS.

DHSS(NI) (1980b) *Report on the Administration of the Health and Personal Social Services in Northern Ireland 1977-79.* Belfast: HMSO.

DHSS(NI) (1982) *Trends in Health and Personal Social Services for 1981.* Belfast: DHSS(NI).

DHSS(NI) (1983a) *Regional Strategic Plan for Health and Personal Social Services in Northern Ireland 1983-87.* Belfast: HMSO.

DHSS(NI) (1983b) *Report on the Administration of the Health and Personal Social Services in Northern Ireland 1980-82.* Belfast: HMSO.

DHSS(NI) (1984) *Mental Health – The Way Forward: Report of the Review Committee on Services for the Mentally Ill in Northern Ireland.* Belfast: HMSO.

DHSS(NI) (1986) *Regional Strategy for the Health and Personal Social Services (NI) 1987-92: Regional Planning Guidelines Manual.* Belfast: DHSS. (January)

DHSS(NI) (1987) *Health and Personal Social Services: A Regional Strategy for Northern Ireland 1987-92.* Belfast: HMSO.

DHSS(NI) (1988) *Trends in Health and Personal Social Services Statistics in Northern Ireland 1987.* Belfast: DHSS

175

DHSS(NI) (1989a) *Working for Patients in Northern Ireland.* Belfast: HMSO. (February)

DHSS(NI) (1989b) *Purchaser and Provider: Implications for relations between Health and Social Services Boards and their directly managed units.* Belfast: HMSO. (November)

DHSS(NI) (1990a) Personal Communication with DHSS(NI).

DHSS(NI) (1990b) *People First: Community Care in Northern Ireland for the 1990s.* Belfast: HMSO.

DHSS(NI) (1990c) *Hospital Statistics 1 April 1989 – 31 March 1990.* Belfast: HMSO.

DHSS(NI) (1991a) *Health and Personal Social Services: A Regional Strategy for Northern Ireland 1992-97.* Belfast: HMSO.

DHSS(NI) (1991b) *Health and Social Services Statistics (NI) 1989-90.* Personal communication with Regional Information office of DHSS(NI).

Dillengburger, Karola (1992) *Violent Bereavement: Widows in Northern Ireland.* Aldershot: Avebury.

Ditch, John (1984) 'Social Security Parity'. *Paper prepared for the Northern Ireland Asembly.* NIA 141-ii, Appendix 11. Belfast: HMSO.

Ditch, John (1988) *Social Policy in Northern Ireland between 1939 and 1950.* Aldershot: Avebury, Gower Publishing Co.

Ditch, John and Morrissey, Mike (1979) 'Recent Developments in Northern Ireland's Social Policy', in M. Brown and S. Baldwin (eds). *The Yearbook of Social Policy.* London: Routledge and Kegan Paul.

Ditch, J., and Morrissey, M. (1992) 'Northern Ireland: Review and Prospects for Social Policy'. *Social Policy and Administration.* Vol 26. No 1 (March). pp. 18-39.

DOH (1991a) *Report on residential accommodation for people who are mentally ill at 31.3.90.* Personal communication with DOH, London.

DOH (1991b) *Report on adult training centres for mentally handicapped people and day centres for mentally ill, elderly and younger physically handicapped people at 31.3.90.* Personal communication with DOH, London.

Dohan, F. C. (1966) 'Wartime changes in hospital admissions for Schizophrenia'. *Acta Psychiatrica Scandinavic.* Vol. 42. pp. 1-23.

Donaldson, Margaret (1983) *The Development of Nursing in Northern Ireland.* D. Phil Thesis. Belfast: University of Ulster at Jordanstown.

Donaldson, S. N. (1975) *Psychiatric Hospitals: Catchment areas and catchment populations.* Belfast: DHSS(NI).

Donaldson, S. N. (1979) *Psychiatric Hospitals in Northern Ireland – a Survey of physical facilities and estimates of future demand.* Belfast: DHSS(NI).

Down (1921-43) *Annual Reports of the Down County Mental Hospital.*

Downshire (1952) *Annual Report of the Downshire Hospital for 1952.*

Dunleavy, P. J. (1980) *Urban Political Analysis.* London: Macmillan Press.

Easton, David (1967) *A Systems Analysis of Political Life.* New York: John Wiley and Sons.

Eire (1927) *Report of the Commission on the Relief of the Sick and Destitute Poor, including the Insane Poor.* Dublin: Government Stationary Office.

Elder, A. T. (1953) 'Health Services of Northern Ireland'. *British Journal of Preventative Social Medicine.* Vol. 7. pp. 105-11.

Eustace, H. J. (1945) 'Addictions under the Mental Treatment Act, Eire 1945'. *Journal of Mental Science.* Vol. 95. July.pp. 693-95.

Evason, E., Darby, J., Pearson, M. (1976) 'Social Need and Social Provision in Northern Ireland'. *Occasional paper in Social Administration.* Coleraine: New University of Ulster.

Finnane, Mark (1981) *Insanity and the Insane in Post Famine Ireland.* London: Croom Helm.

Fisher, M., Newton, C. and Sainsbury, E. (1984) *Mental Health Social Work Observed.* London: Allen and Unwin.

Fitzpatrick, Selwood (1989) *The Special Care Service in Northern Ireland.* MA Thesis. Belfast: QUB.

Flackes, W. D. and Elliot, S., (1989) *Northern Ireland – A Political Directory 1968-88.* Belfast: Blackstaff Press. (First published 1980)

Foucault, Michel (1965) *Madness and Civilization.* New York: Pantheon (Also published in 1967 by Tavistock, London; First published in French in 1961).

Fraser, R. M. (1971) 'The Cost of Commotion: An Analysis of the Psychiatric Sequelae of the 1969 Riots'. *British Journal of Psychiatry.* Vol. 118. pp. 257-64.

Fraser, R. M. *(1974) Children in Conflict.* Middlesex: Penguin Books (First published 1973)

Gaffikin, F. and Morrissey, M. (1990) *Northern Ireland – The Thatcher Years.* London: Zed Books Ltd.

Gelder, M., (1991) 'Adolf Meyer and his influence on British psychiatry' in G. Berrios and H. Freeman (eds). *150 Years of British psychiatry 1841-1991* London: Gaskell and RCPsych. pp. 419-35.

Gibson, J. G. (1957) 'Perspectives in Mental Health'. *Northern Ireland Health Services Conference Papers.* September. (Unpublished papers held at Queen's University Medical Library, Belfast.)

Gibson, Marion (1991) *Order from Chaos : Responding to traumatic events.* Birmingham: Venture Press.

Glover, G. (1989) 'The pattern of admission of Caribbean born immigrants in London'. *Social Psychiatry.* Vol. 24. pp. 49-56.

Goffman, Erving (1961) *Asylums.* New York: Doubleday.

Goffman, Erving (1971) *The Presentation of Self in Everyday Life.* London: Pelican Press. (First published 1959)

Goldberg, D. *(*1978) *Manual of the General Health Questionnaire.* London: NFER-NELSON.

Gostin, Larry (1975) *A Human Condition.* Vol 1. London: MIND, 14 Harley Street, London W1.

Gostin, Larry (1978) *The Mental Health Act 1959: Is it Fair?* London: MIND.

Gostin, Larry (1983) *A Practical Guide to Mental Health Law.* London: MIND.

Graham, N. B. (1932) 'The Mental Treatment Act (NI) 1932: Some practical points'. *Ulster Medical Journal.* Vol. 1. pp. 270-71.

Greer, D. S. (1987) 'The impact of the Troubles on the Law and Legal System of Northern Ireland' in *Northern Ireland: Living with the Crisis,* edited by J. Ward. London: Aldwych Press.

Gregg, Winifred (1990) Mental Health Commissioner (NI). Interview.

Griffiths, Sir Roy (1983) *NHS Management Inquiry Report – together with proceedings of committee and minutes of evidence.* First Report of the House of Commons Social Services Committee Session 1983-84. HC. 209. London: HMSO.

Griffiths, Sir Roy (1988) *Community Care – Agenda for Action.* London: HMSO.

Grob, Gerald (1973) *Mental Institutions in America.* New York: Free Press.

Grob, Gerald (1983) *Mental Illness and American Society,* 1875-1940. New Jersey: Princeton University Press.

Hadden, W., Rutherford, W. and Merrett, J. (1978) 'The injuries of terrorist bombing: a study of 1532 consecutive patients'. *Br. J. Surg.* Vol. 65, pp. 525-31.

Ham, Christopher (1985) *Health Policy in Britain – the politics and organisation of the NHS.* London: Macmillan Ltd. (First published 1982)

Hampson, R. (1986) *Care in the Community: the emerging pattern.* Kent: PSSRU, University of Kent, Paper 393.

Harkness, David (1983) *Northern Ireland since 1920.* Dublin: Helicon Ltd.

HC Deb (1985) *Second Report of the Social Services Committee on 'Community Care with special reference to adult mentally ill and mentally handicapped'.* Session 1984-85. Vol. 1. Paper 13-1. London: HMSO.

HC Deb (1986) *Debate on Draft Mental Health (NI) Order.* Standing Committees. Session 1985-86. Vol. 10, Col. 1-22, 12 March 1986. London: HMSO.

Health Services Manpower Review (1986) *Managing the Transfer for Hospital to Community – with particular reference to mental illness and mental handicap*. Papers of a National Conference. Keele: Adult and Continuing Education Department, Keele University.

Hemphill, R. E. (1941) 'The influence of war on mental disease'. *Journal of Mental Science*. No. 87. pp. 170-82.

Herron, Stanley and Caul, Brian (1992) *A Service for People – Origins and development of the Personal Social Services of Northern Ireland*. Belfast: December Publications.

Herron, Stanley (1990) Social Services Inspector for DHSS(NI). *Personal Interview*.

Heskin, Ken (1980) *Northern Ireland: A Psychological Analysis*. Dublin: Gill and Macmillan.

HHCRU (1991) *Leaving Hospital in Northern Ireland*. Belfast: Queen's University, Health and Health Care Research Unit.

HMSO (1817) *Report of the Select Committee on the Lunatic Poor in Ireland*. HC Sessional Papers Vol. 8. Paper 430.

HMSO (1843) *Report of the Select Committee on the State of the Lunatic Poor in Ireland*. Main Report : HC Sessional Papers Vol. 10. Paper 625. Evidence : HC Sessional Papers Vol. 10. Paper 193.

HMSO (1908) *Report of the Royal Commission on the Care and Control of the Feebleminded 1904-08*. (Radnor Commission) London: HMSO.

HMSO (1909) *Royal Commission on the Poor Laws and Relief of Distress*. Main Report Cd. 4499 (Vol. 37. p. 1) Minority Report Cd. 4499 (Vol. 37. p. 719) Report on Ireland Cd. 4630 (Vol. 38. p. 1) London: HMSO.

HMSO (1918) *Annual Report of the Board of Control for England and Wales*. London: HMSO.

HMSO (1926) *Report of the Royal Commission on Lunacy and Mental Disorder 1924-26 (Macmillan Commission)*. Cmd. 2700. London: HMSO.

HMSO (1942) *Social Insurance and Allied Services* (Beveridge Report). Cmnd. 6404. London: HMSO.

HMSO (1944) *A National Health Service*. White Paper. Cmnd. 6502. London: HMSO.

HMSO (1946) *Second White Paper on the National Health Service*. Cmd. 6761. London: HMSO.

HMSO (1951) Ministry of Health. *Report of the Committee on Social Workers in the Mental Health Services* (Mackintosh Report). Cmd. 8260. London: HMSO.

HMSO (1956) Ministry of Health. *Report of the Committee of enquiry into the cost of the National Health Service* (Guillebaud Committee). Cmd. 9663. London: HMSO.

HMSO (1957) *Report of the Royal Commission on the Law relating to Mental Illness and Mental Deficiency 1954-57* (Percy Commission). Cmnd. 169. London: HMSO.

HMSO (1959) Ministry of Health. *Report of the Working Party on Social Workers in the Local Authority Health and Welfare Services* (Younghusband Report). London: HMSO.

HMSO (1962) *Hospital Plan for England and Wales.* London: HMSO.

HMSO (1968a) *Administrative Structure of the Medical and related services in England and Wales.* Green Paper from the Ministry of Health. London: HMSO.

HMSO (1968b) *Report of the Committee on Local Authority and Allied Personal Social Services* (Seebohm Report). Cmnd. 3703. London: HMSO.

HMSO (1969) *Text of communiqué following discussions between the United Kingdom government and the Northern Ireland government in October 1969.* Cmnd. 4178. London: HMSO.

HMSO (1970) *The Future Structure of the NHS.* Second Green Paper from the Ministry of Health. London: HMSO

HMSO (1972) *Report of the Tribunal appointed to enquire into the events on Sunday, 30 January 1972, which led to loss of life in connection with the procession in Londonderry on that day* (Widgery Report). London: HMSO.

HMSO (1975a) *Better Services for the Mentally Ill.* White Paper. Cmnd. 6233. London: HMSO.

HMSO (1975b) *Report of a Committee to consider, in the context of civil liberties and human rights, measures to deal with terrorism in Northern Ireland* (Gardiner Report). Cmnd. 5847. London: HMSO.

HMSO (1975c) *Report of the Committee on Mentally Abnormal Offenders* (Butler Report). Cmnd. 6244. London: HMSO.

HMSO (1976) *White Paper on Public Expenditure 1975/76 to 1979/80.* Cmnd. 6393. London: HMSO.

HMSO (1978) *A Review of the Mental Health Act 1959.* Cmnd. 7320. London: HMSO.

HMSO (1979) *Report of the Royal Commission on the National Health Service* (Merrison Report). Cmnd. 7615. London: HMSO.

HMSO (1985) *Government response to the Second Report from the Social Services Committee (1984-85 Session) 'Community Care with special reference to adult mentally ill and mentally handicapped people.'* Cmnd. 9674. London: HMSO.

HMSO (1986) *Making a Reality of Community Care.* Report of the Audit Commission for Local Authorities (England and Wales). London: HMSO.

HMSO (1988) *Working for Patients.* White Paper. Cm. 555. London: HMSO.

HMSO (1989) *Caring for People – Community care in the next decade and beyond.* White Paper. Cm. 849. London: HMSO.

HMSO(Irl) (1874) *Twenty third report on District, criminal and private lunatic asylums in Ireland.* Dublin: HMSO.

HMSO(Irl) (1904) *Statutory Rules and Orders Revised to December 1903.* Vol. 8. pp. 44-45. Dublin: HMSO.

HMSO(Irl) (1921) *69th Report of the Inspectors of Lunatics (Irl) for the year 1919.* Cd. 1127. Dublin: HMSO.

HMSO(NI) (1924) *Report of the Inspectors of Lunatics (NI) for 1921 and 1922.* Cmd. 28. Belfast: HMSO.

HMSO(NI) (1926) *4th Report of the Inspectors of Lunatics (NI) for the year 1925.* Cmd. 68. Belfast: HMSO.

HMSO(NI) (1927) *Report of the Departmental Commission on Local Government Administration in Northern Ireland 1924-27* (Johnstone Report). Cmd. 73. Belfast: HMSO.

HMSO(NI) (1930a) *Report on the Administration of the Home Office Services of the Ministry of Home Affairs for the year 1929.* Cmd. 120. Belfast: HMSO.

HMSO(NI) (1930b) *Northern Ireland Index to Statutory Rules and Orders in force on 31 August 1930.* Belfast: HMSO.

HMSO(NI) (1931) *Report of the Committee on the Financial Relations between the State and Local Authorities* (Leslie Committee). Cmd. 131. Belfast: HMSO.

HMSO(NI) (1933) *Report on the Administration of the Home Office Services of the Ministry of Home Affairs (NI) for the year 1932.* Cmd. 155. Belfast: HMSO.

HMSO(NI) (1944) *Select Committee on the Health Services in Northern Ireland* (Stevenson Committee). House of Commons (NI) Paper 601. Belfast: HMSO.

HMSO(NI) (1946) *Mental Deficiency in Northern Ireland. Report of the Mental Health Committee of the Northern Ireland Health Advisory Council* (Gordon Committee). Belfast: HMSO.

HMSO(NI) (1948a) *Report on the Administration of the Ministry of Health and Local Government (NI) for the period 1 April 1938 to 31 December 1946.* Cmd. 258. Belfast: HMSO.

HMSO(NI) (1948b) *The Future Mental Health Services of Northern Ireland: An explanatory memorandum on the Mental Health Act (NI) 1948.* Issued by the Ministry of Health and Local Government. Belfast: HMSO.

HMSO(NI) (1948c) *Report on the Administration of Home Office Services (NI) 1939-46.* Cmd. 262. Belfast: HMSO.

HMSO(NI) (1951) *Report on Health and Local Government Administration in Northern Ireland during the period 1 January 1947 to 31 December 1949*. Cmd. 288. Belfast: HMSO.

HMSO(NI) (1952) *Report on Health and Local Government Administration in Northern Ireland for the year 1950*. Cmd. 303. Belfast: HMSO.

HMSO(NI) (1954) *Report on Health and Local Government Administration in Northern Ireland for the year 1952*. Cmd. 320. Belfast: HMSO.

HMSO(NI) (1955a) *Report on Health and Local Government Administration in Northern Ireland for the year 1953*. Cmd. 332. Belfast: HMSO.

HMSO(NI) (1955b) *Report of the Committee on the Health Services in Northern Ireland 1954-55* (Tanner Report). Cmd. 334. Belfast: HMSO.

HMSO(NI) (1956) *Report on Health and Local Government Administration in Northern Ireland for the year 1955*. Cmd. 359. Belfast: HMSO.

HMSO(NI) (1957a) *Report of the Committee on the Finances of Local Authorities* (Nugent Committee). Cmd. 369. Belfast: HMSO.

HMSO(NI) (1957b) *Report on Health and Local Government Administration in Northern Ireland for the year 1956*. Cmd. 379. Belfast: HMSO.

HMSO(NI) (1958) *Report of the Advisory Committee on Child Guidance and Speech Therapy* (Main Report). Belfast: HMSO.

HMSO(NI) (1959) *Report on Health and Local Government Administration in Northern Ireland for the year 1958*. Cmd. 406. Belfast: HMSO.

HMSO(NI) (1961) *Report on Health and Local Government Administration in Northern Ireland for the year 1960*. Cmd. 429. Belfast: HMSO.

HMSO(NI) (1962) *Report on Health and Local Government Administration in Northern Ireland for the year 1961*. Cmd. 444. Belfast: HMSO.

HMSO(NI) (1963) *The Belfast Regional Survey and Plan* (Matthew Report). Cmd. 451. Belfast: HMSO.

HMSO(NI) (1964) *Report on Health and Local Government Administration in Northern Ireland for 1962 and 1963*. Cmd. 474. Belfast: HMSO.

HMSO(NI) (1967) *The Re-shaping of Local Government: Statement of Aims*. Cmd. 517. Belfast: HMSO.

HMSO(NI) (1969a) *The Re-shaping of Local Government: Further Proposals*. Cmd. 530. Belfast: HMSO.

HMSO(NI) (1969b) *Disturbances in Northern Ireland* (Cameron Report). Cmd. 532. Belfast: HMSO.

HMSO(NI) (1969c) *The Police in Northern Ireland* (Hunt Report). Cmd. 535. Belfast: HMSO.

HMSO(NI) (1969d) *The Administrative Structure of the Health and Personal Social Services in Northern Ireland*. Green Paper. Belfast: HMSO.

HMSO(NI) 1970 *Report of the Review Body on the Administration of Local Government in Northern Ireland* (Macrory Report). Cmd. 546. Belfast: HMSO.

HMSO(NI) (1971) Ministry of Health and Social Services (NI) *Consultative Document on the Re-structuring of the Personal Health and Personal Social Services in Northern Ireland.* Belfast: HMSO.

HMSO(NI) (1972) *Violence and Civil Disturbances in Northern Ireland in 1969* (Scarman Report). Cmd. 566. Belfast: HMSO.

HMSO(NI) (1973) *Northern Ireland Annual Abstract of Statistics.* Belfast: HMSO.

HMSO(NI) (1981) *Northern Ireland Review Committee on Mental Health Legislation* (MacDermott Committee). Belfast HMSO.

Hoggett, Brenda (1990) *Mental Health Law.* London: Sweet and Maxwell. (First published 1984)

Holywell (1952) *Annual Report of Holywell Hospital for 1952.*

Hoyle, J. S. and Hawkesworth, T. S. (1956) *Mental Health Officers guide to the Lunacy and Mental Treatment Acts.* Leeds: Elsworth Bros. Ltd.

Hunter, Richard and Macalpine, Ida (eds) (1982) *Three Hundred Years of Psychiatry* 1535-1860. New York: Carlisle Publishing Inc. (First published 1963)

Illich, Ivan (1975) *Limits to Medicine.* London: Marion Boyers.

Isles, K. S. and Cuthbert, N. (1957) *An Economic Survey of Northern Ireland.* Belfast: HMSO.

ITO (1960-63) *Reports of the Industrial Therapy Organisation.* Downpatrick: ITO.

Johnson, D. S. (1985) 'The Northern Ireland Economy 1914-39', in L. Kennedy and P. Ollerenshaw (eds) *An Economic History of Ulster 1820-1940. pp. 184-223.* Manchester: University Press.

Jones, Katherine (1973) *The development of the Hospital Services of Northern Ireland : an annotated guide to the literature.* Thesis for a Fellowship of the Library Association.

Jones, Kathleen (1960) *Mental Health and Social Policy 1845-1959.* London: Routledge and Kegan Paul.

Jones, Kathleen (1972) *A History of the Mental Health Services* 1744-1971. London: Routledge and Kegan Paul.

Jones, Kathleen (1988) *Experiences in Mental Health – Community care and social policy.* London: Sage Publications.

Jones, Kathleen (1991a) 'The culture of the mental hospital' in G. Berrios and H. Freeman (eds). pp. 17-28.

Jones, Kathleen (1991b) 'Law and mental health: sticks or carrots?' in G. Berriod and H. Freeman (eds). pp. 89-102.

Jones, Kathleen (1992) *Personal Communication.*

Jones, K., Brown, J. and Bradshaw, J. (1984) *Issues in Social Policy.* London: Routledge and Kegan Paul. (First published 1978)

Jones, K. and Fowles, A. J. (1984) *Ideas on Institutions.* London: Routledge and Kegan Paul.

Jones, Maxwell (1968) *Beyond the Therapeutic Community*. Yale: University Press.

Kay, Adah and Legg, Charlie (1986) 'Discharged to the Community – a review of housing and support in London for people leaving psychiatric care.' London: GPMH publications.

Kee, M., Bell, P., Loughrey, G., Roddy, R., Curran, P. (1987) 'Victims of Violence: A Demographic and Clinical Study'. *Med. Sci. Law*. Vol. 27. No. 4. pp. 241-47.

Kennedy, Liam and Ollerenshaw, Philip (eds) (1985) *An Economic History of Ulster 1820-1940*. Manchester: University Press.

Klein, Rudolf (1974) 'Social Policy and Public Expenditure'. Bath: University, Centre for Studies in Social Policy.

Klein, Rudolf (1983) *The Politics of the National Health Service*. London: Longman. (Politics Today Series)

King, D., Mc Meekin, C., Elmes, P. (1977) 'Are we as depressed as we think we are?' *Ulster Medical Journal*. Vol. 46. pp. 105-12.

King, D., Griffiths, K., Reilly, P. and Merrett, D. (1982) 'Psychotropic drug use in Northern Ireland 1966-80: Prescribing trends, inter- and intra-regional comparisons and relationship to demographic and socioeconomic variables.' *Psychological Medicine*. Vol. 12. pp. 819-33.

Kirkpatrick, T. P. (1931) *A Note on the History of the care of the insane in Ireland up to the end of the Nineteenth Century*. Dublin: University Press.

Kittrie, N., (1971) *The Right to be Different : Deviance and enforced therapy*. Baltimore: John Hopkins University Press.

Laing, R. D. (1960) *The Divided Self: An Existential Study in Sanity and Madness*. London: Tavistock.

Lawrence, R.J. (1965) *The Government of Northern Ireland: Public Finance and Public Services 1921-64*. Oxford: Clarendon Press.

Leaper, R. R. (1931) *'Presidential Address to the Royal Medico Psychological Association'*. *J. Ment. Sc*. Vol. 77 (Oct). pp. 683-91.

Lewis, A. (1941) 'Incidence of neurosis in England under war conditions'. *Lancet*. Vol. 2. pp. 175-83.

Loughrey G. C. and Curran, P. S. (1987) 'The psychopathology of civil disorder' in Dawson, A. and Besser, G. (eds) *Recent Advances in Medicine* No. 20. pp. 1-17. London: Churchill Livingstone.

Loughrey, G. C., Bell, P., Kee, M., Roddy, R. J. and Curran, P. (1988) 'Post-Traumatic Stress Disorder and Civil Violence in Northern Ireland'. *British Journal of Psychiatry*. Vol. 153. pp. 554-60.

Lukes, S. (1974) *Power: A Radical View*. London: Macmillan.

Lyons, H. A. (1971) 'Psychiatric sequelae of the Belfast riots'. *British Journal of Psychiatry*. Vol. 118. pp. 265-73.

Lyons, H. A. (1972) 'Depressive Illness and Aggression in Belfast'. *British Medical Journal.* Vol. 1. pp. 342-44.

Mac Donald, Michael (1981) *Mystical Bedlam.* New York: Cambridge University Press.

Malcolm, Elizabeth (1989) *Swift's Hospital.* Dublin: Gill and Macmillan.

Malcolm, Elizabeth (1988) *Women and Mental Illness in nineteenth century Dublin.* Belfast: Queen's University. Institute of Irish Studies. (Paper delivered in January)

Martin, A. R. (1935) 'Recent trends in psychiatry'. *Ulster Medical Journal.* Vol. 4. pp. 146-52.

Mc Cartan, William (1963) *'Mental Health in Northern Ireland – laws ancient and modern.' Mental Health.* Vol. 22. pp. 12-16.

Mc Clelland, Roy (1988) 'The Madhouses and Mad doctors of Ulster'. *Ulster Medical Journal.* Vol. 57. No. 2. Oct. pp. 101-20.

MHC(NI) (1988) *First Biennial Report of the Mental Health Commission (NI) 1986-88.* Belfast: MHC(NI)

MHC(NI) (1990) *Information Leaflet of the Mental Health Commission (NI).* Belfast: MHC(NI)

MHC(NI) (1991) *Second Biennial Report of the Mental Health Commission (NI) 1988-90.* Belfast: MHC(NI)

MHRT(NI)(1992) Mental Health Tribunal (NI) *Personal Communication.*

Mill, John Stuart (1910) *Utilitarianism, Liberty and Representative Government.* Everyman edition, London: J. M. Dent and Sons. (First published 1859)

MIND (1977) *Evidence to the Royal Commission on the NHS with regard to services for mentally ill people.* London: MIND. (March)

MIND (1978) *A New Deal for Mental Patients: MIND's further evidence to the Royal commission on the NHS.* London: MIND.

MIND (1983) 'Care in the Community: Keeping it local.' *Report of the 1983 Annual Conference.* London: MIND.

Moore, Michael (1984) *Law and Psychiatry.* New York: Cambridge University Press.

Morris, R., Woods, R., Davies, K., Morris. W.(1991) 'Gender differences in carers of dementia sufferers.' *British Journal of Psychiatry.* Vol. 158 (Supplement 10). pp. 69-74.

Morrissey, Mike and Ditch, John (1982) 'Social Policy implications of emergency legislation in Northern Ireland.' *Critical Social Policy.* Vol. 1. Issue 3. pp. 19-39.

Mulligan, J., Robinson, C., Casement, E., (1964) 'A survey of psychiatric services in Northern Ireland hospitals'. *Report to the Northern Ireland Hospitals Authority.* Belfast: NIHA.

Murray-Parkes, Colin (1975) 'Whatever becomes of redundant world models – a contribution to the study of adaptation to change. *Brit. Journal Med. Psychology.* Vol. 48. pp. 131-37.

New Ireland Forum (1984) *Final Report.* Dublin: Government Stationary Office.

NIA (1985a) Northern Ireland Assembly. *Report prepared for the Debate on the Draft Mental Health (NI) Order.* NIA 205. Belfast: HMSO.

NIA (1985b) Northern Ireland Assembly. *Debate on Draft Mental Health (NI) Order.* Official Assembly Report. Vol. 16. No. 12 & 13. Belfast: HMSO.

NIAMH Minutes (1959-64) *Minutes of committee meetings of the Northern Ireland Association for Mental Health.* Belfast: NIAMH.

NIAMH (1984) *Mental Health Statistics for Northern Ireland.* Belfast: NIAMH.

NIHA (1948-73) *Annual Reports of the Northern Ireland Hospitals Authority.* (Numbers 1-25 and Final Report). Belfast: NIHA.

NIHA (1954b) *Report of the NIHA committee on hospital and specialist services (*Corbett Committee). Belfast: NIHA.

NIHC Deb (1932) *Debate on the Mental Treatment Bill.* Vol. 14. Cols. 547, 600, 1189, 1190, 1533, 1542, 1550. Belfast: HMSO.

NIHC Deb. (1944) *Budget Speech.* Vol. 27, Session 1944-45, Col. 1252. Belfast: HMSO.

NIHC Deb. (1948) *Debate on the Mental Health Bill (NI) 1948.* Vol. 32, Cols. 1994, 2083, 2457, 2680, 2685, 2709, 2725. Belfast: HMSO.

NIHC Deb. (1961) *Debate on the Mental Health Bill (NI) 1961.* Vol. 48. Session 1961. Cols. 1410, 2047, 2629, 3140, Vol. 50. Session 1961-62. Cols. 164, 378.

NI Sen Deb. (1932) *Debate on the Mental Treatment Bill (NI) 1932.* Vol. 14. Col. 177, 231, 265, 295, 316.

NI Sen Deb. (1948) *Debate on the Mental Health Bill (NI) 1948.* Vol. 32. Col. 265, 268, 295, 311, 324.

NI Sen Deb. (1961) *Debate on the Mental Health Bill (NI) 1961.* Vol. 45. Col. 515, 605, 708, 759, 794, 812, 840.

O'Donnell, Owen (1989) *Mental Health Care Policy in England: Objectives, Failures and Reforms.* York: Centre for Health Economics. (Paper 57)

O'Hare, Aileen and Walsh, Dermot (1985) *Activities of Irish Psychiatric Hospitals and Units 1985.* Dublin: The Health Research Board.

O'Leary, C., Elliot, S. and Wilford, R.A. (1988) *The Northern Ireland Assembly 1982-86: A Constitutional Experiment.* London: Hurst.

O'Malley, P. P. (1969) 'Attempted Suicide before and after the communal violence in Belfast, August 1969: A Preliminary Study'. *Journal of the Irish Medical Association.* Vol. 65. pp. 109-13.

Parkinson, R. E. (1969) *The Centenary of Downshire Hospital.* Downpatrick: no publisher.

Parry-Jones, William (1972) *The Trade in Lunacy.* London: Routledge and Kegan Paul.

Patten, Chris (1984) *Paper delivered to a meeting of health care professionals and administrators.* Belfast: Queen's University. (14 November)

Paykel, E. S. (1991) 'Depression in Women'. *British Journal of Psychiatry.* Vol. 158. Supplement 10. pp. 22-29.

Pilkington, Francis (1939) 'Facilities for Mental Treatment: Past and Present'. *Irish Journal of Medical Science.* No. 161. May. pp. 193-208.

Pilling, Steve (1983) 'The Mental Health (Amendment) Act 1982: Reform or cosmetics?'. *Critical Social Policy.* Vol. 3. Issue 7. pp. 90-96.

Pilowsky, L., O'Sullivan, G. et al (eds) (1991) 'Women and Mental Health – Papers of the Women and Mental Health International Conference'. *British Journal of Psychiatry.* Vol. 158. Supplement 10.

Pines, Malcolm (1991) 'The development of the psychodynamic movement' in G. Berrios and H. Freeman (eds) *150 Years of British Psychiatry 1841-1991.* pp. 206-301. London: Gaskell and Royal College of Psychiatrists.

Platt, S. (1984) 'Unemployment and suicidal behaviour: a review of the literature'. *Social Science and Medicine.* Vol.19. pp. 93-115.

Porter, Roy (1987) *Mind-Forged Manacles,* London: Athlone Press.

Powell, J. E. (1961) *Speech by the Minister of Health, the Rt. Hon. Enoch Powell.* Report of the Annual Conference of the National Association for Mental Health. London: NAMH.

Prior, Pauline (1992a) 'The Approved Social Worker – Reflections on Origins'. *BJSW* Vol. 22. pp. 105-19.

Prior, Pauline (1992b) *Northern Ireland Mental Health Services: Bibliography and Chronology.* Occasional Paper in Social Policy. York University: SPSW.

PRO(NI) CAB 4/513   *N. Ireland Cabinet meeting 19 June 1942.*

PRO(NI) CAB 4/642   *N. Ireland Cabinet meeting 15 Nov. 1945.*

PRO(NI) CAB 9A/3/1   *Financial Situation (1924-30).*

PRO(NI) CAB 9B/176/1 *Government grants to mental hospitals in Northern Ireland 1930-47.*

PRO(NI) CAB 9B/179   *The Lodge Inebriate Retreat (1930).*

PRO(NI) CAB 9B/256   *Child Guidance Clinic (1942-46).*

PRO(NI) CAB 9C/48/1   *Beveridge Report (1942-56).*

PRO(NI) D 1022/2/22   *Paper on financial relations between Northern Ireland and Great Britain – written by Sir Ernest Clarke.* (circa. 1926)

PRO(NI) HOS 14/1/2/1   *Downshire Mental Hospital Management Committee – Minutes of meetings April 1916 to March 1919.*

PRO(NI) HOS 14/1/2/2 – as above April 1919 to March 1922.

PRO(NI) HOS 14/1/2/3 – as above April 1922 to March 1925.

PRO(NI) HOS 14/1/2/5 – as above April 1928 to March 1931.

PRO(NI) HOS 28/1/1/13 *Belfast (Purdysburn) Mental Hospital Management Committee, Minutes of meetings 1917-21.*

PRO(NI) HOS 28/1/1/14 – as above for the period 1921-25.

PRO(NI) HOS 28/1/1/15 – as above June 1925 to August 1929.

PRO(NI) HOS 28/1/1/16 – as above Sept. 1929 to Dec. 1933.

PRO(NI) HSS 16/2/26 *Mental Health Services Committee (1945-48).*

PRO(NI) HSS 16/3/104 *Health Services Bill, Mental Health and Deficiency Services – Policy and Progress (1946-47)*

PRO(NI) HSS 16/3/125 *Pre-frontal leucotomy in Northern Ireland (1946-55)*

PRO(NI) HSS 16/4/26 Nursing Establishments in mental hospitals (Reports by Nursing Officer and Mental Nurses Committee 1947-50)

PRO(NI) HSS 16/4/52 *Functions of an almoner (1947)*

PRO(NI) HSS 16/4/79 *Mental Health Bill, Recommendations of the Mental Health Services Committee (1947)*

PRO(NI) HSS 16/5/70 *Mental Health Bill, Consultations with interested Bodies (1948)*

PRO(NI) HSS 16/5/107 *Mental Hospitals: Report on survey of present accommodation and proposals for modernisation and future developments (1947-49)*

PRO(NI) HSS 16/5/150 *NIHA Special Care colony (1948)*

PRO(NI) HSS 16/5/151 *Special Care Institutions (not Muckamore) (1948)*

PRO(NI) HSS 16/5/174 *Tuberculosis and infectious diseases in mental hospitals (1947-57)*

PRO(NI) HSS 16/6/156 *Mental Health Act (NI) 1948: Mentally infirm persons (1948-57)*

Purdysburn (1950) *Annual Report for Purdysburn Hospital, Belfast for 1952.* Belfast: NIHA.

Raftery, James (1985) 'Health Services North and South', *Administration* No. 33 Part 3. Dublin: Institute of Public Administration.

Regional Hospitals Council (NI) (1944) *Survey of the Hospital Services On Northern Ireland.* Belfast: Regional Hospitals Council (NI).

Regional Hospitals Council (NI) (1946) *The Red Book: A Plan for the Hospital Services of Northern Ireland.* Belfast: Regional Hospitals Council (NI).

Reid, G.H. (1958) 'Northern Ireland Mental Health Services'. *The Hospital.* February. pp. 113-19.

Riessman, F. Cohen, J. Pearl, A. (eds) (1964) *Mental Health of the Poor.* New York: The Free Press.

Robertson, G. (1931) 'Mental Out-patients clinics'. *Journal of Mental Science.* Vol. 77. January. pp. 22-52.

Robins, Joseph (1986) *Fools and Mad: A History of the Insane in Ireland.* Dublin: Institute of Public Administration.

Robinson, C. B.(1950) 'The problem of the aged in mental hospitals'. *Ulster Medical Journal.* Vol. 19. pp. 5-11.

Rose, Richard (1971) *Governing Without Consensus – An Irish perspective.* London: Faber and Faber Ltd.

Rose, Richard (1987) *Ministers and Ministries: A functional analysis.* Oxford: Clarendon Press.

Rothman, David (1971) *The Discovery of the Asylum – Social Order and Disorder in the New Republic.* Boston, Mass: Little, Brown and Co.

Rothman, David (1980) *Conscience and Convenience – The Asylum and its Alternatives in Progressive America.* Boston, Mass: Little, Brown and Co.

Royal College of Physicians of London (1944) *Second Interim Report of the Committee on Psychological Medicine.* London: RCPhys.

Royal College of Psychiatry (1977) 'Comments on the Review of the 1959 Mental Health Act'. London: *Psychiatric Bulletin.* January. pp. 9-18.

RMPA (1945) *Memorandum on the Future Organization of the Psychiatric Services.* London: Royal Medico-Psychological Association. (Joint Report with the BMA and RCPhys.)

Royal Ulster Constabulary (1990) *Chief Constable's Annual Report 1989.* Belfast: Police Authority.

Scheff, Thomas J. (1966) *Being Mentally Ill.* London: Weidenfeld and Nicholson.

Scull, Andrew (1979) *Museums of Madness: The Social Organization of Insanity in Nineteenth Century England.* London: Allen Lane.

Scull, Andrew (1984) *Decarceration: Community Treatment and the Deviant.* Oxford: Polity Press. (First published 1977).

Scull, Andrew (1985) 'Madness and Segregative Control' in Phil Brown (ed) *Mental Health Care and Social Policy. pp. 17-40.* London: Routledge and Kegan Paul.

Scull, Andrew (1989) *Social Order/Mental Disorder – Anglo American Psychiatry in Historical Perspective.* London: Routledge.

Scull, Andrew (1991) 'Psychiatry and its historians'. *History of Psychiatry.* Vol. 2. Part 3. No. 7.

Sedgwick, Peter (1982) *Psycho Politics.* London: Pluto Press.

Sheppard, M. (1990) *Mental Health: The Role of the Approved Social Worker.* Sheffield: JUSSR, Sheffield University in collaboration with Community Care.

Shiell, Alan and Wright, Ken (1988) *Counting the Costs of Community Care: Mental Handicap.* University of York: Centre for Health Economics.

Showalter, Elaine (1987) *The Female Malady – women, madness and English culture 1830-1980*. London: Virago Press. (First published 1985)

Simpson, John (1983) 'Economic Development: Cause or Effect in the Northern Ireland Conflict' in Darby, J. (ed) *Northern Ireland: The Background to the Conflict*. Belfast: Appletree Press.

Skultans, Vieda (1979) *English Madness: Ideas on Insanity 1580-1890*. London: Routledge and Kegan Paul.

Strain, R. W. M. (1967) 'The History of the Ulster Medical Society'. *Ulster Medical Journal*. Vol. 36. No. 2. pp. 73-110.

Szasz, Thomas (1961) *The Myth of Mental Illness*. New York: Harper and Row.

Szasz, Thomas (1970) *Manufacture of Madness*. New York: Harper and Row.

Szasz, Thomas (1987) *Insanity: The Idea and its Consequences*. New York: John Wiley and Sons.

Thompson, C. (ed) *(1987) The Origins of Modern Psychiatry*. Chichester: John Wiley & Sons.

Thompson, J. (1989) 'Deprivation and Political Violence in Northern Ireland 1922-85'. *Journal of Conflict Resolution*. Vol. 33 No. 4. pp. 676-99.

Thornicroft, G. (1991) 'Social deprivation and rates of treated mental disorder – developing statistical models to predict psychiatric service utilisation'. *British Journal of Psychiatry*. Vol. 158. pp. 475-84.

Tyrone and Fermanagh (1950) *Annual Report of the Tyrone and Fermanagh Mental Hospital*.

Ulster Year Book 1926, 1929, 1932, 1935, 1938, 1947, 1950, 1957-59. Belfast: HMSO.

Unsworth, Clive (1987) *The Politics of Mental Health Legislation*. Oxford: Clarendon Press.

Walker, Nigel (1980) *Punishment, Danger and Stigma*. Oxford: Basil Blackwell.

Walsh, B. (1990) 'The future of Psychiatric Services in Ireland'. *The Irish Journal of Psychiatry*. Autumn. pp. 5-11.

Wansbrough, N. and Miles, A. *(1969) Industrial Therapy in Psychiatric Hospitals*. A Kings Fund Report Supplement. London: King Edward's Hospital Fund.

Warr, P. (1987) *Work, Unemployment and Mental Health*. Oxford: University Press.

Webster, Charles (1991) 'Psychiatry and the early NHS: the role of the Mental Health Standing Committee', in G. E. Berrios and H. Freeman (eds) pp. 103-16.

Weir, T. W. H. (1949) 'Legislation and Mental Health in Northern Ireland'. *Journal of Mental Science*. Vol. 95. July. pp. 673-84.

Wichert, Sabine (1991) *Northern Ireland since 1945*. London: Longman.

Williams, John (1990) *The law of Mental Health*. London: Fourmat Publishing.

Williamson, Arthur (1970) 'The Beginnings of State Care for the Mentally Ill in Ireland'. *Economic and Social Review*. January. pp. 281-90.

Williamson, Arthur (1992) Mental Health Commissioner (NI). *Personal communication*.

Wilson, Tom (1989) *Ulster: Conflict or Consent*. Oxford: Basil Blackwell.

Windlesham, Lord (1973) 'Ministers in Ulster: The machinery of Direct Rule'. *Public Administration*. Vol 51. Part 3. pp. 261-72.

Wright, Ken (1988) *Cost Effectiveness in Community Care*. University of York: Centre for Health Economics. Paper 33.

Wright, T. D. (1989) Acting Director Nurse Education, Belfast. *Personal Interview*.

Index

hospitals
Individual: Downshire 10, 19, 22, 49-51, 76, 80, 85; Gransha 76; Holywell 81, 85; Purdysburn 10, 19, 23, 39, 47, 51, 76; St Lukes 16, 134; Tyrone and Fermanagh 17, 76; Mater 80, 104
beds 67, 70, 134-6
Hospital Plan 1962 78
hostels 74, 80, 114, 138-9, 143, 153
Health and Personal Social Services
Regional Strategies 118, 120, 122, 137, 140
restructuring 110-4

Industrial Therapy
Organization 151
Ireland 87, 138, 164
Irish Asylums Workers
Union 20

Jones, Kathleen 3, 38

legislation
mental health 24-5, 62-3, 87, 91-2, 126-34
National Insurance Act (NI) 1946 62
Welfare Services Act (NI) 1949 93
lunacy 25-6; criminal 23-4, 30
Inspectorate (NI) 12-15, 19, 51

Maconaghie, Bessie 90, 93
Macrory Review Body 111
MacDermott Committee 127-31
Malcolm, Elizabeth 7
Mental Health Commission (NI) 132
Mental Health Review Tribunal (NI) 92, 132

Northern Ireland
Assembly 117, 129
Northern Ireland regional organizations
Association for Mental Health 87, 93, 130, 139
Civil Rights Association (NICRA) 98
Health Advisory Council 59-60
Hospitals Authority 74-6, 84-7, 113
Regional Hospitals Council 59-60
Tuberculosis Authority (NITA) 62
nurses 20, 68, 81-2, 146, 156

O'Malley, Dr Pierce 80, 104

PARR 118, 121
PESC 114
political violence 98, 102
Pollock, Hugh 12, 45, 52
psychopathy 119, 121

RAWP 118, 121
Republic of Ireland : *see* Ireland
Robins, J. 7
Royal Medico Psychological Association (RMPA) 36, 68
Royal Commission
on Lunacy and Mental Disorder (1924-26) 33-4
on Mental Illness and Mental Deficiency (1954-57) 87, 123
on the National Health Service 119

Scull, Andrew, 5-6, 165
Select Committee on the Health Services (NI) 57, 59, 68